Karima BENABDELLAH
Chabha MEGHNI
Fatma KESSAL

Final dissertation

Karima **BENABDELLAH**
Chabha **MEGHNI**
Fatma **KESSAL**

Final dissertation

Study of BCR/Abl molecular transcript
quantification at diagnosis and follow-up of CML
patients

ScienciaScripts

Imprint

Any brand names and product names mentioned in this book are subject to trademark, brand or patent protection and are trademarks or registered trademarks of their respective holders. The use of brand names, product names, common names, trade names, product descriptions etc. even without a particular marking in this work is in no way to be construed to mean that such names may be regarded as unrestricted in respect of trademark and brand protection legislation and could thus be used by anyone.

Cover image: www.ingimage.com

This book is a translation from the original published under ISBN 978-620-6-69803-6.

Publisher:
Sciencia Scripts
is a trademark of
Dodo Books Indian Ocean Ltd. and OmniScriptum S.R.L publishing group

120 High Road, East Finchley, London, N2 9ED, United Kingdom
Str. Armeneasca 28/1, office 1, Chisinau MD-2012, Republic of Moldova, Europe
Printed at: see last page
ISBN: 978-620-7-63615-0

Contents

General introduction

Chronic myeloid leukëmia (CML) is a malignant hëmopathy belonging to the group of myeloproliative syndromes (MPS) [1]. It is characterisedërisëe by the presence of a chromosomal abnormality affecting hëmatopoiëtic cells, this abnormality is due to a balanced reciprocal translocation t (9; 22) (q34; q11) leading to the formation of the Philadelphia chromosome (Ph1).

To this end, this translocation leads to a specific fusion gene called BCR-Abl. The BCR-Abl fusion protëin has high tyrosine kinase enzyme activity.

Molecular monitoring of bcr-abl transcript levels by quantitative PCR is increasingly usedë to ë assess patient response to therapy. This has become intëressant to Гёre of imatinib when residual disease falls below the detection threshold of conventional cytogënëtics.

This approach makes it possible to introduce the concept of major or complete molecular remission (MMR or CMR), which is much more sensitive than cytogënëtic response. It allows molecular monitoring of the disease under Tyrosine Kinase Inhibitor (TKI) treatment and, consequently, adjustment or substitution of TKIs in the event of ineffectiveness confirmed by monitoring of BCR/Abl transcripts.

Studies have been carried out on the impact of BCR/ABL molecular transcript quantification in the diagnosis and follow-up of patients with CML, such as the South African [2] and Nigerian [3] studies, which showed a MMR of 50% in patients followed up for 24 months or more.

In Algeria, diagnostic resources (conventional cytogenetics) and molecular monitoring (RT-PCR) are still inadequate or even non-existent. As a result, numerous difficulties are encountered on a daily basis in the rapid and effective management of patients.

Finally, due to a lack of data on a national scale, we thought it would be useful to carry out a retrospective study on 30 CML patients treated with TKIs and who had benefited from BCR/Abl transcript monitoring, in order to determine whether there was a relationship between the quantification of the BCR/Abl molecular transcript and the therapeutic response.

Summary bibliography

Chapter I: Presentation of Chronic Myeloid Leukemia.

1. History

1840: The first descriptions of cases of chronic myeloid leukaemia (CML), first by A. Donne, then by J.H. Benett and R. Virchow. Studying patients with dëcëdës, they noted a link between the clinical signs, splenomegaly and hepatomegaly, and the blood, which they described as "suppurating" or even "white blood". [4]

1846: The first case of diagnosis in a living patient is written by Fuller, and the term "leucocythaemia" is proposed in 1848.

In 1870, Neumann asserted that the cells responsible for this pathology originated in the bone marrow. [5]

1951: the concept of myëloprolifërative syndrome (MPS) was first developed by W. Dameshek.

In 1960, discovery of the first chromosomal marker correlated with a ^oplastic pathology by Nowell and Hungerford called the "Philadelphia chromosome" in rëfërence to its dëovery. [6]

In 1973, J. Rowley discovered the reciprocal translocation and ëquilibrëe between the long arm of chromosome 9 and the long arm of chromosome 22, the t (9; 22) (q34; q11). This translocation corresponds to the Philadelphia chromosome. [7]

1985: identification of the BCR-ABL1 fusion gene and the p210 BCR- ABL1 fusion protëin (implicated in the pathophysiology of CML). [8]

In 1998, an anti-tyrosine kinase drug [imatinib (Glivec)] was marketed, which acts precipitously on the **bcr-abl1** protëin[9].

We report on the major milestones in the evolution of CML treatment:

2006: Dasatinib was granted marketing authorisation as a second-line treatment for chronic-phase CML.

2007: Nilotinib was granted marketing authorisation as a second-line treatment for chronic-phase CML and iiccx'Drees (but not blast-crisis CML).

2008: the WHO has given a new classification to SMP with a new name: "myëloprolifëractive iK'opDsmes".

2010: Dasatinib and nilotinib received marketing authorisation for first-line treatment of chronic-phase CML, following the publication of two multicentre phase III trials. [10]

2013 : The European Commission dëlivrë a marketing authorisation nmirclK' for bosutinib valid throughout the European Union. [11]

2. Epidemiology of CML

Chronic my'loid leukëmia is a rare disease, its incidence in the world varies depending on the country, the lowest incidence is 0.7 foundëe in Sweden and China, the highest is 1.7 foundëe in Switzerland and the United States. [12]

In France, approximately ten new cases of CML per year have ëlë reported' per million inhabitants, or 600 new cases per year. [13]

It occurs in 2-5% of childhood leukaemias and 7-15% of adult leukaemias. The median age at diagnosis is 50 years. In adults, the average age is between 30 and 60, with a peak between 40 and 50.

This disease mainly affects men, with a sex ratio close to 2: between 1.4 and 2.2 men are affected for every woman. There is a higher excess mortality rate for men during the first four years, after which the involution becomes similar for both sexes. [14]

The survival rate in developed countries is twice that in developing countries. This may be due to the lack of treatment or the difficulty of accessing care in these countries.

In Algeria, according to a study by Professor Ahmed Nacer in 2010 [15]:
- The incidence is rising in Algeria, from 0.19 in 1994 to 0.40 in 2004 and 0.44 in 2009.
- The overall incidence rate for the period 1994-2009 is 0.34/100,000.
- The specific incidence rate for the over-14s in 2009 was 0.69
- There was a slight male predominance, with a sex ratio of 1.01.
- The average age at diagnosis is 43.5, with a peak between 36 and 45, making CML a disease of young adults.

However, the absence of a national register means that the incidence of this disease can only be assessed approximately.

3. Etiological factors :

In the vast majority of cases, no etiology is found.

However, people chronically exposed to benzene and patients treated with chemotherapeutic agents or immunosuppressants appear to be at risk of developing CML. [16]

Exposure to ionising radiation could also play a favourable role. This hypothesis, suggested by the increased incidence of CML in survivors of the Hiroshima atomic bomb, is supported in vitro by the increased frequency of detection of the BCR-Abl rearrangement after irradiation of initially BCR-ABL-negative cell lines. [17]

4. Pathophysiology of CML

CML is a hematopoietic stem cell cancer. The initial chronic phase is manifested by excessive myeloid production in the bone marrow, mainly involving the granulocytic line. At this stage, there is no leukemic hiatus and no significant peripheral blastosis.

The discovery of the Philadelphia chromosome, observable in cytogenetics, demonstrated for the first time that a chromosomal anomaly could be associated with a cancerous disease, in this case leukaemia. The Philadelphia chromosome is the expression of the *BCR/Abl* chimeric gene encoding an oncogenic protein of the same name. It is an acquired reciprocal translocation between chromosome 9 and chromosome 22. The formulation of this translocation is as follows: t (9;22) (q34;q31). [18]

4. 1 Pathogenesis

The purpose of this translocation is to shorten the long arm of one of the two chromosomes 22, known in cytogenetics as the "Philadelphia chromosome". The fusion protein resulting from this translocation will lead to leukaemic transformation **(Fig. 1).** The BCR/Abl protein activates various cell signalling pathways.

The hematological consequences are manifold: increased cell proliferation, altered cell adhesion properties, inhibition of apoptosis, degradation of regulatory proteins, altered DNA repair.

The BCR/ABL protein has high tyrosine kinase enzyme activity.

The SH1 domain that carries this activity is dependent on the energy supplied by 1 ATP.

Control of phosphorylation is crucial for cellular homeostasis. Abnormal tyrosine kinase activity will have disastrous consequences.

The BCR/Abl fusion protein exists in two conformations, inactive and active.

In the active conformation, the activation loop opens after ATP binding and forms a support for the substrate, which can then be phosphorylated.

This precise aspect is the basis of the pharmacological research that has led to the development of specific inhibitors of tyrosine kinase activity.

The effects of these drugs as ATP competitors block the ATP binding site, maintaining the BCR/Abl protein in an inactive conformation with no phosphorylation activity **(Fig. 2)**. [18]

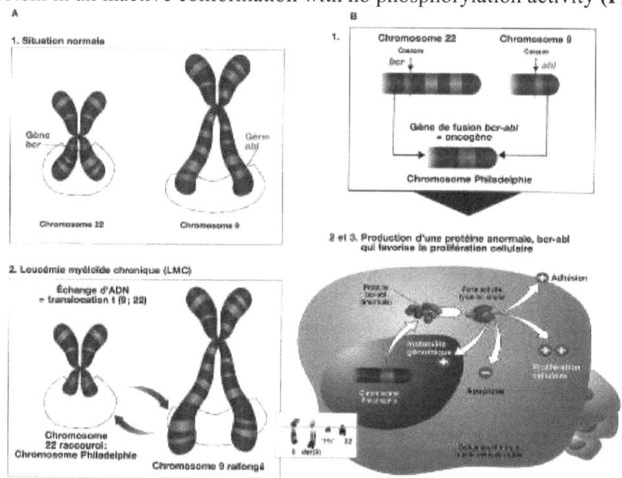

Figure 1: Pathogenesis of chronic myeloid leukaemia. **a:** CML: an exchange of DNA between two chromosomes in bone marrow stem cells; **b:** appearance of the abnormal fusion gene[18].

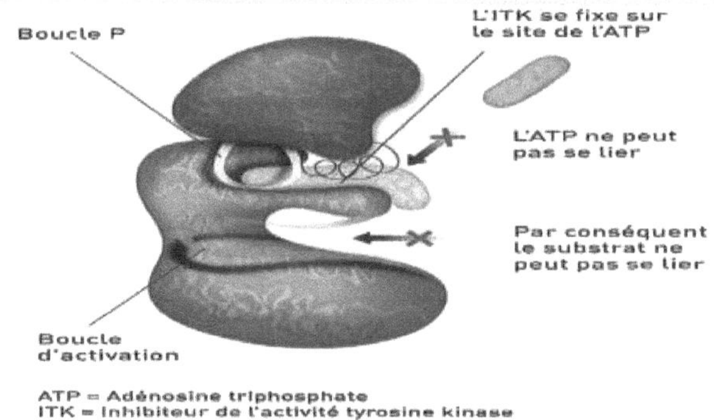

Figure 2: Mode of action of tyrosine kinase inhibitors (TKIs)[18].

4.2 Genes involved in translocation and their cellular consequences

4.2.1 *ABL* gene and its protein

The Abelson oncogene (*c-ABL*) is located on chromosome 9 at position 9q34. [19] There are two possible variants for the first exon, 1a and 1b, and the messenger RNAs produced measure 6 and 7 kb respectively. Two variëtës of protëins of approximately 145 kDa are synthesised depending on the first exon, 1a or 1b. [20] The protëin containing exon 1b is "myristoylated" (i.e. modified by a saturated fatty acid lipid group on a glycine residue), which results in its localisation to the plasma membrane. The absence of this glycine residue in form 1a (the majority) results in predominantly nucIear localisation. In the nuclear compartment, Abl acts as a negative regulator of the cell cycle. During the G0 phase, Abl binds to DNA and forms a complex with cycle-inhibiting proteins such as pRb (retinoblastoma protein). During the G1/S transition, the protëine pRb is phosphorylated and dissociates from Abl, allowing it to be activated. When localized in the cytoplasm, the Abl protein plays a role in cell growth and proliferation, participating in signal transduction initiated by certain growth factor receptors.

4. 2. 2 *BCR* gene and its protein

The *BCR* gene, located on the long arm of chromosome 22, was discovered by cloning the so-called *major-breakpoint cluster region* (M-BCR). It extends over 135 kb, comprises 23 exons and allows the transcription of two types of messenger RNA with molecular weights of 4.5 and 6.7 kb respectively, which encode a 160 kDa protëin with ubiquitous expression. [21]

4 .2. 3. BCR-ABL gene and fusion protein

The most common rearrangements found in CML are the fusion products of the *ABL* gene broken between exons 1 and 2 and the *BCR gene* broken in a region where the breakpoints are variable, known as M-BCR (Major BCR).

There are other variants of the t (9;22) translocation, most of which are responsible for different leukaemic phenotypes. Mention should be made of the e1a2 fusion, resulting from a break in the m-BCR (*minor* BCR), i.e. between exons 1 and 2 of *BCR*. It produces a 190 kDa chimeric protein whose tyrosine kinase activity is more intense than that of the 210 kDa protein. This molecular variant is mainly found in Philadelphia chromosome-positive lymphoblastic leukaemia. Another variant, which includes a *BCR* gene interrupted in the l-BCR (*micro-BCR*), between exons 19 and 20, enables the synthesis of a 230 kDa chimeric protein. The latter molecular form is thought to correspond to slowly progressive haemopathies marked by moderate neutrophil hyperleukocytosis, with or without thrombocytosis. [22] **(Fig. 3).**

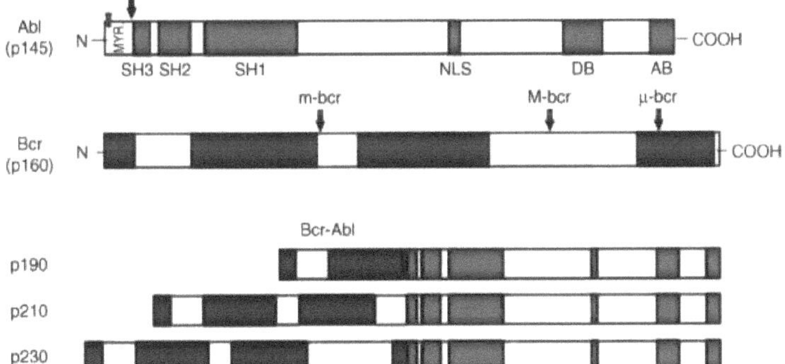

Figure 3. Bcr-Abl protein variants as a function of breakpoints. Different breakpoints in the *BCR* gene lead to the synthesis of three different protein variants[13].

The physiological protein tyrosine kinase Abl is tiutoregulated physically, i.e. by conformational modification. Fusion with BCR modifies this auto-inhibition and permanently activates the kinase.

4.   2.4 Intracellular signalling pathways leading to leukemogenesis

The phosphorylation of a very large number of substrates is responsible for the properties of the leukëmic cell, which distinguish it from a normal cell. In fact, self-activation and loss of regulation of tyrosine kinase activity lead to the direct or indirect activation and recruitment of signalling pathways involved in the processes of proliferation, apoptosis, différenciation and cell adhesësion. **(Appendix I)**

Mechanisms of action of the fusion protein :

The Bcr-Abl protein induces phosphorylation of a very large number of substrates, which is responsible for the properties of the leukaemia cell **(Appendix I).**

This excessive phosphorylation activates different cell signalling pathways. This will have multiple consequences at hematological level:

-    Altered adhesion properties of immature tumour cells to medullary stroma and extracellular matrix.

-    Activation of mitotic signals by induction of a proliferative and anti-apoptotic signal. - Inhibition of apoptosis.

-    Degradation of proteins by the proteasome. These proteins include those involved in DNA repair, which could partly explain the genetic instability of BCR-Abl positive leukaemia cells.

-    Genomic or genetic instability and the appearance of very intense mutational activity. [18,23, 24 ,]

A study of the intracellular pathways responsible for cell self-renewal showed that the progenitors of patients in blast phase could self-renew, a property that exclusively concerns the stem cell. [25]

Chapter II: Positive diagnosis of CML

1. Clinical presentation

The natural history of CML comprises three evolving phases: *a first phase known as "chronic"*, pauci symptomatic, followed by a *second phase,* caractërisëe by an *acceleration of* the disease, and finally a *third phase,* appelëe *"acute transformation"*, taking the appearance of a secondary ;iiguc' leucëmia, resistant or refractory to treatment, leading to the patient's dëcës.

1.1. Clinical study of the disease in the chronic phase:

1.1.1. Circumstances of discovery:

The slow and insidious development explains why CML is discovered fortuitously in the presence of splënomëgalia or riiemogram disturbances. [26]

More rarely, the disease may be discovered on the occasion of an inaugural complication such as venous thrombosis, gout attack, splenic infarction, visual disturbances, or respiratory failure due to leukostasis. [27,28, 29]

1.1.2. Clinical examination :

Many patients are asymptomatic or only mildly symptomatic at this stage. № Nevertheless, three major syndromes may be encountered:

-    An alteration in general condition, Hëc a hyper metabolism, associating astlK'nie, emaciation, and more rarely, fëbricule and sweating.

-    A tumour syndrome, largely caractërisë by a splënomëgalie.

-    Signs of leukostasis, in particular priapism, are now quite exceptional. [30]

The main symptoms found are : [30,31, 32]

General signs :

-    AstlK'nie : a 83

-    Weight loss: a 61

-    Fever: a 11

Signs associated with splenomegaly :

-    Splënomëgalie : 50% to 70

-    Hëpatomëgalia: 48%.

-    Abdominal pain: a 33

2. Biological diagnosis :

2.1. Blood count

I . The haemogram is the clë examination, as it alone can suggest the diagnosis of CML.

Hyperleukocytosis, anaemia and thrombocytosis are the blood anomalies most frequently encountered.

Hyperleukocytosis was marked, ranging from 20,109 to 500,109 leukocytes/L. The mean leukocytosis is 120.10^9 leukocytes/L (N: 4-10 G/L or $4-10.10^9$ leukocytes/L), predominantly neutrophils (30% to 40%), with a more discreet eosinophilia (5% to 10%) and a more marked basophilia (3% to 10%)['28].

Myelogenesis (i.e. the passage of myeloid cells at all stages of differentiation into the blood) is constant and harmonious, with no hiatus in differentiation, consisting of metamyelocytes,

myelocytes and some promyelocytes and, more rarely, myeloblasts. [30]

Anemia (normocytic and normochromic) is uncommon and moderate.

Thrombocytosis is common, often exceeding 500,000/mm3.

Sometimes very high, it is rarely responsible for thrombotic events due to associated thrombopathy. [30]

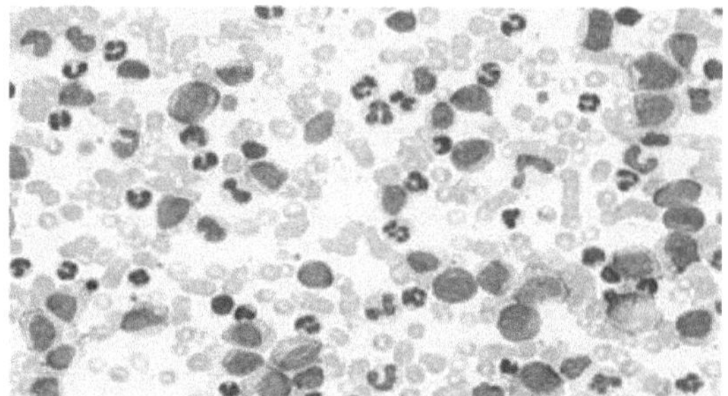

Figure 4: Blood smear: CML in chronic phase: hyperleukocytosis (100 Giga/l): neutrophil polynucleosis and myelmania. [26]

However, diagnostic tests cannot be limited to blood tests: a bone marrow sample is essential, firstly to confirm whether CML is chronic or not, on the basis of the criteria for bone marrow blast infiltration, and secondly to carry out cytogenetic tests.

2.2. Myelogram :

It confirms the myeioproliferative syndrome by showing an extremely rich marrow, made up mainly of granular cells which are myelocytes, metamyelocytes and polynuclear cells, with all stages of maturation represented (absence of maturation hiatus), and medullary blastosis of less than 10% in the chronic phase.

As in the blood, basophilia and even eosinophilia may be found. Megakaryocytes are often increased in number and small in size. The percentage of erythroblasts and lymphocytes is very low.

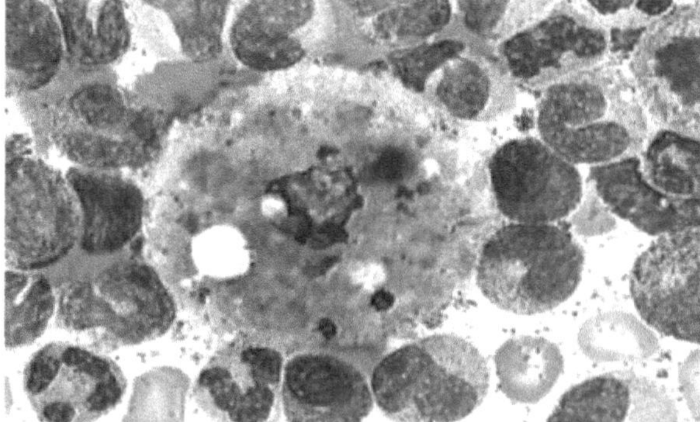

Figure 5. myëlogram of a patient with chronic-phase CML: sea-blue histiocyte. [26]

Occasionally, overload histiocytic cells are seen, resulting from an accumulation of glycolipids from excessive leukocyte destruction. Although the myelogram is not useful for diagnosing CML, it can be used to confirm the stage of the disease and to perform the initial karyotype. [26, 30,33]

2.3. Bone biopsy:

Unnecessary for the diagnosis of CML. The appearance of fibrosis is one of the signs of acceleration of the disease. [30]

2.4. Cytogenetic tests :

2.4.1. Conventional cytogenetics: the karyotype

It is an essential test for the diagnosis of CML and is performed on a mëdullary sample, or on a blood sample if myëlëmia is significant. [34]

Karyotyping reveals the **Ph** chromosome in 95% of cases, and detects additional karyotypic abnormalities to the Ph chromosome that may be present at diagnosis, or appear during disease progression, and which appear to have an impact on patient outcome and the quality of response to treatment. [35]

It can also be used to assess the cytogenetic response by determining the percentage of residual Ph1+ cells. [30 ,36]

In 5% of cases, the BCR-Abl fusion gene results from either: a complex variant translocation, involving one 3ёте or even several chromosomes, or a cryptic insertion of chromosomal material, undetectable by conventional cytogdndtic techniques.

In this case, CML is said to be ***Ph negative***, BCR-Abl positive, and only ***Fluorescence In Situ Hybridization (FISH) and molecular biology (RT-PCR)*** techniques will allow detection of the hybrid gene and the BCR-ABL transcript (RNA) respectively. [37]

2.4.2. Molecular cytogenetics: FISH

FISH is a targeted examination which does not visualise the whole genome; it highlights the **BCR-Abl** fusion signal in nuclei (interphase FISH) and mitoses (metaphase FISH), particularly in the case of ***Ph1 negativity*** (masked Ph1). It reveals cryptic abnormalities (insertions, micro deletions of the long arm of ddrivd 9).

It is thought to be more sensitive than conventional karyotyping for monitoring therapeutic response (better definition of complete cytogdndtic response) and to correlate better with molecular response. However, it does not reveal additional cytogdndtic abnormalities. [30,37]

FISH is not systematically recommended to diagnose CML or to assess its cytogenetic response to treatment, but it remains essential in the case of ***Ph-negative, BCR-Abl positive*** CML (5% of cases) where conventional karyotyping does not reveal the Ph chromosome. It can sometimes be a useful complement when the number of metaphase cells (blood or medullary) obtained is insufficient or even absent. [38,39]

2.4.3. Molecular biology tests :

The fundamental diagnostic criterion is the presence of the *BCR-Abl* fusion gene, detected by molecular biology.

> ***Reverse transcriptase polymerase chain reaction*** (RT-PCR):

Detects the Bcr-Abl fusion transcript in medullary cells or, more easily, from a blood sample taken in a simple ethylene diamine tetra-acetic acid (EDTA) counting tube, even after 36 hours at room temperature.

RT-PCR is a qualitative test that can identify bcr-abl fusion RNA (ribonucleic acid) with extreme sensitivity. This technique shows that more than 50% of patients with negative cytogenetics are in fact bcr/abl+. [40]

> ***Real-Time Quantitative PCR (RT-Q-PCR)*** :

This test is carried out on medullary or blood cells [41], and enables the BCR-Abl fusion transcript to be detected and quantified, as well as revealing the molecular subtype produced. It is a good tool for diagnosing and monitoring the progression of CML, and for assessing the molecular response to treatment]. [13,18]

RQ-PCR based on detection of the fluorescence generated by amplification: the fluorescence is proportional to the quantity of transcript present in the sample to be analysed [42].

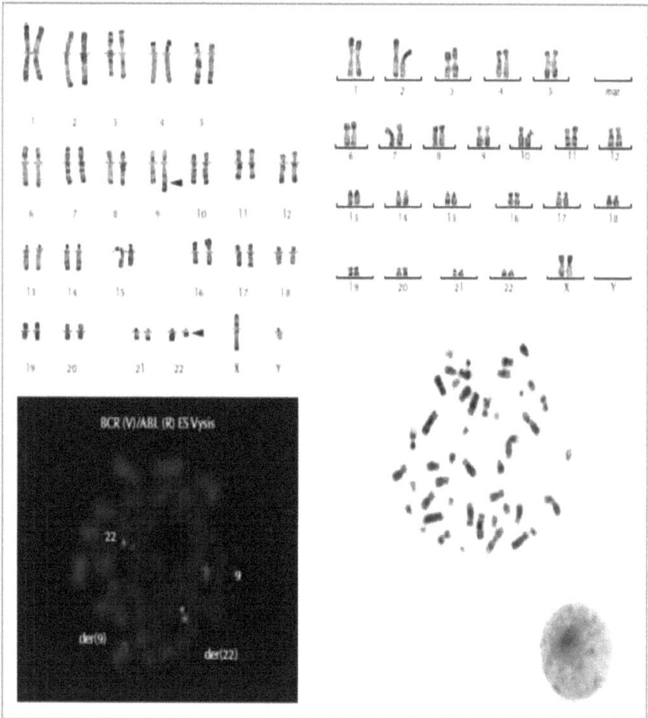

Figure 6. Karyotype and *fluorescent in situ hybridisation* (FISH) of two patients with CML. On the left, the classic Philadelphia chromosome is seen and the fusion is confirmed by FISH. On the right, the karyotype is normal, but FISH clearly shows a fusion of *BCR* and *Abl*: this is a Philadelphia chromosome masked by an imbalanced translocation. [43]

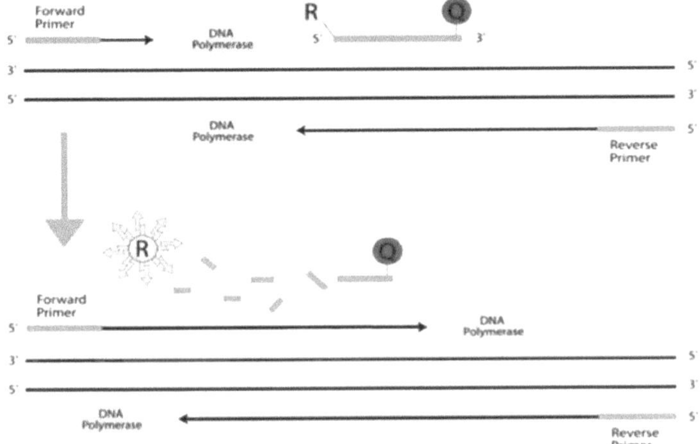

2.4.4. 7. BCR-ABL amplification: R = fluorochrome ёteКеиг "reporter";
Q = suppressor fluorochrome "quencher"[43].

2.5. Other biological tests:

- I Ivperuricx'mia and hyperuraturia are common.
- Vitamin B12 levels are high, correlated with hyperleukocytosis.
- Sëric and urinary lysozyme can be ёкуё.
- Functional testing of platelets showed acquired thrombopathy.
- Cultures of hëmatopoiëtic progënitors show an increase in pluripotent and granulomonocytic precursors. These progënitors are ёalso found in ёкуё numbers in the blood. [40]

3.   Differential diagnosis :

3.1. The chronic phase:

Before the t(9;22) translocation is demonstrated by cytogënëtic analysis (karyotype) or by demonstration of the BCR-Abl fusion transcript by molecular biology, the differential diagnoses are those of hyperleukocytosis associated with myëlëmia. [44]

- **Reactionary myeloma:**

They are secondary to infection, often severe, corticotherapy or mëdullary mëtastases. They are characterised by the absence of circulating blasts and low numbers of promyelocytes. In contrast, no Ph chromosome is ever observed [44].

- **Other myeloproliferative disorders** :
- **Myeloid splenomegaly or primary myelofibrosis** :

It most commonly develops in subjects aged over 60, and is characterised by iyperleukocytosis with myeloma, and above all by erythroblastosis in the blood, leading to the characteristic erythromyeloma. The marrow is subject to varying degrees of fibrosis, making it difficult to perform a myelogram. The Philadelphia chromosome is never found on cytogenetic analysis. [33]

- **Essential thrombocythemia** :

It is characterised by significant thrombocytosis with moderate hyperleukocytosis. This is a diagnosis of elimination; other myeloproliferative syndromes must be ruled out by the absence of a Philadelphia chromosome. No myelofibrosis (primary myeloid splenomegaly) and no increase in blood mass (polycythemia vera). [43]

- **Vaquez disease or primary polycythemia :**

Diagnosis is based on increased total blood volume, splenomegaly and myeloid hyperplasia with erythroblastic predominance. The karyotype shows the absence of the Philadelphia chromosome. [43]

- **chronic myelomonocytic leukemia :**

This is probably one of the most difficult differential diagnoses: it is a borderline entity between myeloproliferative syndrome and myelodysplastic syndrome.

There is hyperleukocytosis with myelhemia, the characteristic feature of which is monocytosis (more than 1000 elements/mm3). Cytological signs of myelodysplasia are also present. The diagnosis of CML can be excluded by the absence of the Philadelphia chromosome and especially by the absence of the BCR-Abl fusion transcript in molecular biology [44].

3.2. The acute phase:

Ph-chromosomal acute lymphoblastic leukëmia is a differential diagnostic problem with acute transformation-phase CML of lymphoi de phënotype. While the presence of splënomëgalia and myëlëmia associated with basophilia points more towards a diagnosis of accutised CML, only the karyotype performed during remission after induction chemotherapy will allow a decision to be made, showing in the case of accutised CML the persistence of the Ph chromosome in all the metaphases analysed [44].

4. Complications frequently observed :

4.1. Thrombocytosis

It accompanies any myeloproliferative syndrome, and can be the cause of venous thrombosis and haemorrhage, sometimes revealing the disease.

Thrombocytopenia is possible and increases the risk of haemorrhage.

4.2. Leukostasis

It is due to hyperleukocytosis, and can cause acute respiratory insufficiency. Fundus may show leukemic retinitis.

4.3. Hyperuricemia

This is a consequence of hyperleukocytosis, and can manifest itself as gout attacks or nephritic colic.

Chapter III: Phases of CML progression and prognostic prognostic scores

1. Evolutionary phases of CML

Chronic myeloid leukëmia evolves in three phases: the chronic phase, the acceleration phase, and the phase of transformation into acute leukëmia.

1.1. The chronic phase

This premiëre phase is progressive in onset; it lasts an average of 4 to 5 years. Clinical signs are often insidious and many patients are asymptomatic at the time of diagnosis, suspected in the face of a hëmogram гeяHзë systëmatically (40% of cases). However, three main syndromes may be encountered:

- an alteration in the general state of health, linked to hypermetabolism, associating asthenia, weight loss and, more rarely, a fëbricule and sweating;
- a tumour syndrome, largely characterised by splenomegaly (50%), sometimes responsible for digestive symptoms;
- signs of leukostasis, in particular priapism, are now quite exceptional.

1.2. Accelerated phase :

It corresponds to the transition between the chronic phase and the blast phase. It lasts 12 to 18 months on average. However, it may be virtually non-existent, in which case the blast phase ëis "explosive" (around 20% of cases). The World Health Organisation (WHO) has defined clinical and biological crores of acceleration, which narrowly precede the blast phase refractory to any treatment (**Table I**). [45]

Table I: Clinicobiological criteria for acceleration according to the International Bone Marrow Transplant Registry (IBMTR).

• Leukocytosis difficult to control with conventional treatment: hydroxyurea or busulfan
• Rapid doubling of white blood cell count (5 days)
• Presence of more than 10% blood or bone marrow blasts
• Presence of more than 20% blasts + blood or medullary promyelocytes
• Presence of more than 20% basophilic or eosinophilic blood cells
• Anemia or thrombocytopenia not due to treatment
• Persistent thrombocytosis
• Additional cytogenetic abnormalities
• Sudden increase in splenomegaly
• Development of myelofibrosis or chloroma
• Patient in chronic phase but who has had a blast crisis

Tableau II.   WHO definition of disease progression [46].

Features	WHO
Blood or medullary blasts(%)	10-19
Blood basophilia (%)	>20
Paquettes($*10^9$ /L)	<100 (thrombocytosis not related to treatment) Or > 1000 (persistent thrombocytosis, not sensitive to treatment)
Cytogenetics	Clonal evolution
Other	Splenomegaly and number of leukocytes not sensitive to treatment

2.3. Acute phase or blast crisis :

It occurs with a median age of 4 years and is defined by the presence of more than 20% medullary blasts or more than 30% blood or medullary blasts and promyelocytes.

It is accompanied in дёпёгаl by an increase in the clinical signs of acceleration (alteration of the general state, splenomegaly, anemia, thrombopenia, medullary fibrosis) and sometimes by its own symptomatology: fidvre, hdpatomdgalia, adenopathies and bone pain.

Like any acute leukaemia, it may be accompanied by a tumour syndrome and signs of medullary insufficiency. Extramedullary blastic localisations may also be seen, including meningeal involvement or soft tissue chloromas. Two-thirds of cases are myeloblastic and one-third lymphoblastic.

Tableau III.   Criteria for diagnosis of blast phase according to the WHO [47].

Features	WHO
Blood or mëdullary blasts	>20 %
Blast proliferation	Extra-medular
Bone biopsy	Large foci of blasts
Remarks	70% AML and 30% ALL

2. Prognostic scores :

The positive diagnosis is completed by an evaluation of the severity criteria, integrated into prognostic scores calculated and valid on cohorts of patients.

Sokal score

The best known of these, the Sokal score [48], was established on a cohort of patients treated with interferon in 1984. It has subsequently been validated for other treatments.

Its parameters include the patient's age, the size of the spleen, the number of platelets and the number of blood blasts. It defines three levels of risk of progression to transformation: low, intermediate and high.

Hasford score

In 1998, Hasford's score [49] ёlё dëveloppë de ташёге to integrate in addition to the prëcëdents two other paramëtres likely according to the literature to impact prognosis: these are the percentage of basophils and eosinophils in the blood count. The same risk levels are defined.

EUTOS score

To simplify matters, the EUTOS score was published in 2011 by *the European Leukemia Net group* [50]: it depends solely on blood basophilia and the size of the spleen on clinical examination.

The sum of these two parameters affected by coefficients defines the patient's probability of not having a competitive cytogenetic response (CCyR) at 18 months of treatment.

Patients are therefore considered to be at high risk if their EUTOS score is above 87.
These three prognostic scores have therefore been developed in the context of different
treatments, and their significance depends on the treatment instituted. However, the Sokal
score is still the most widely used in practice, even though it predates current therapies.
A logarithmic calculation based on these independent prognostic factors gives an index value
for each patient. See **Table IV** for details of the prognostic crores of the different scores and
the formulae for calculating the indices.

Table IV. Prognostic criteria for the different scores and formulae for
calculating the indices

Hasford	The risk	Sokal
< 780	Low	< 0,8
> 780 - < 1 480	Intermediary	0,8 -1,2
> 1 480	Student	> 1,2

Sokal score (> 45 years) = EXP(0.011*(age-43.4) + 0.0345*(rate-7.51) +
0.188*(platelets/700)**2-0.563) + 0.0887*(blasts-2.1)

Sokal score (< 45 years) = EXP(0.0255*(rate-8.14) + 0.0324*(blasts-
2.22) + 0.1025*(platelets/700)**2-0.627)-0.0173* (hematocrit - 34.2)-
0.2682*(gender-1.40)

Score of
Hasford = (0.6666*age + 0.042*rate + 0.0584*blasts + 0.0413*eosinophils +
0.2039*basophils + 1.0956*platelets)* 1 000

with: age = 0 if < 50 years, or = 1 otherwise; basophils = 0 if < 3%.
or = 1 otherwise platelets = 0 if < 1500 x 10^9 /L or = 1 otherwise

Hasford	The risk	Sokal
< 780	Low	< 0,8
> 780 - < 1 480	Intermediate	0,8 -1,2
> 1 480	Student	> 1,2

Chapter IV: Treatment of CML

CML has long ële been a disease with no curative treatment, chemotherapy only being symptomatic.

However, the 1980s saw the emergence of new treatments, such as INF-a, which improved the overall survival of patients.

Therapeutic progress in CML has been dramatic over the past decade with the introduction of imatinib mesylate (IM) [51]. The specific, targeted action of this agent has necessitated a complete revision of the principles of monitoring and treating the disease at all stages.

In this section, we describe the different CML treatments and the levels of response obtained.

1. Conventional chemotherapy :

1.1 Busulfan

Busulfan is an alkylating agent used at a dose of 0.1 mg/kg/day. Complete hematological responses have been obtained in 23-54% of cases, but very rare major cytogenetic responses have been reported (1-2.5%) [52]. This therapy is known for its delayed and long-lasting hematological toxicity, predominantly affecting polynuclears [53]. Busulfan was abandoned after the discovery of hydroxyurea [54].

1.2 . Hydroxidee

Hydroxyurea (Hydrea) is the least harmful treatment, resulting in haematological remission in around 70% of cases. However, cytogenetic remission is very rare. Hydroxyurea is prescribed at a dosage of 40 mg/kg/day, and is a ribonucleotide reductase inhibitor, reducing DNA synthesis. It results in complete hematological remission in 39% to 53% of cases, with less severe adverse effects than busulfan. [53]

Today, hydroxyurea is only useful in cases of symptomatic hyperleukocytosis, or thrombocytosis in excess of 1000 Giga/l. It is also indicated in cases of limited life expectancy or intolerance to other therapies. [30]

2. Hematopoietic stem cell allograft

Conventional or attenuated conditioning allograft transplantation is still the only curative treatment dëmontrë for CML [55]. However, despite the progress made in reducing the toxicity and mortality associated with transplantation, it is still accompanied by a non-negligible mortality rate, which limits its indications. There is general agreement that allograft transplantation should be avoided as a first-line treatment in chronic phases where no treatment has been given, except for young patients under 20 years of age with a low risk score for transplantation (Gratwohl score) [56]. On the other hand, in advanced phase, allogeneic transplantation is still appropriate in cases of non-response or failure to respond to tyrosine kinase inhibitors, or in cases of BCR-ABL T315I mutation in particular. [57]

3. Interferon alpha :

This has been the standard treatment since 1980.

INF-a is a cytokine with antiproliferative action on normal and tumour cells. INF <<interferes" with the immune system but its mechanism of action in CML remains largely unknown. It produces hematological responses in 50-80% of cases [58] and also cytogenetic

responses in 20-50% of cases. [59]

4. Tyrosine kinase inhibitors :

The revolution in the management and prognosis of CML patients came in 1998 with the advent of the first tyrosine kinase inhibitor (TKI), *imatinib mesylate*, which was granted marketing authorisation in France in 2001.

TKIs are competitive ATP antagonists, more or less specific for the chimeric tyrosine kinase characteristic of CML. They prevent phosphorylation of its substrates and therefore activation of the cell survival and expansion mechanisms underlying the leukaemic process *(figure 8)*.

4.1 First-generation tyrosine kinase inhibitors :

— Imatinib Mesylate (STI571) or GLivec® (GLivec®)

Imatinib (Glivec®, Novartis), administered as imatinib mesylate, is a 2-phenylaminopyrimidine developed by Brian Druker and his colleagues at Ciba-Geigy in Switzerland in the early 1990s. [60]

Firstly пошшё STI571 (*signal transduction inhibitor* 571), this is an ITK with sëlective affinity for the *BCR-Abl* kinase, as well as for the two variants of the platelet dërivë growth factor receptor PDGF-R and for CD117 (membrane receptor encodedë by the *c-KIT* gene*)*.

Mechanism of action :

It is based on the neutralisation of the tyrosine kinase activity of the BCR/ABL protëine by competitive inhibition of ATP at its catalytic site.

The result is inhibition of autophosphorylation, proliferation and induction of apoptosis.

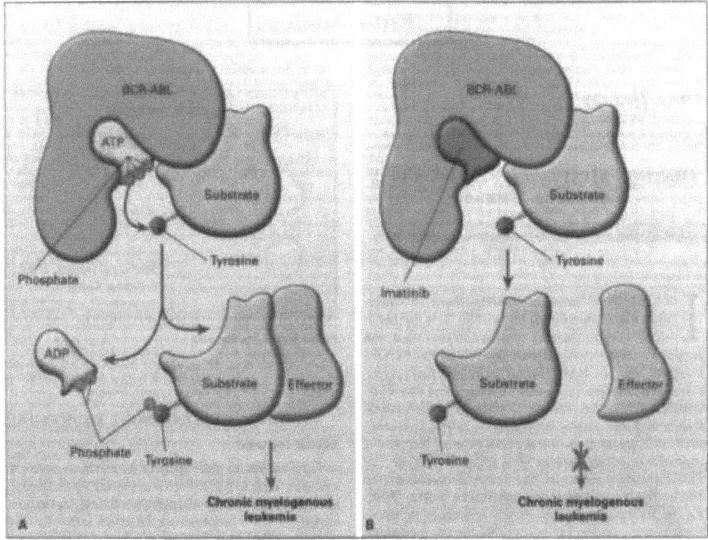

Figure 8: Mechanisms of action of imatinib mesylate. [61] (See BCR-ABL protëin and its tyrosine kinase activity).

-Left: BCR /Abl oncoprotein, with the ATP binding site: the substrate is phosphorylated on a tyrosine residue, enabling it to activate other effector molecules.

-Right: imatinib occupies the ATP site, inhibiting the action of ATP and therefore the phosphorylation of the substrate.

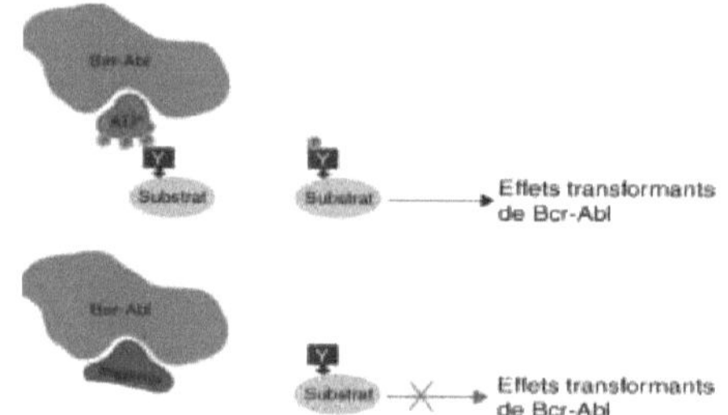

Figure 9: Mechanism of action of imatinib. Imatinib competes with adenosine triphosphate (ATP) at the tyrosine kinase domain of Abl. Blockade of the catalytic site leads to inhibition of phosphorylation of target substrates[61].

Pharmacokinetics :

Its oral bioavailability is 98%, allowing virtually complete absorption.

Maximum concentration is obtained in 2 to 4 hours. [62]

Its tissue distribution is high, and its metabolism in the liver is intense.

Its elimination and metabolism are predominantly biliary, with great pharmacokinetic variability between individuals due to multifactorial factors. [63]

Dosage :

It varies according to the stage of the disease:

— Chronic phase: 400 mg/d in a single dose, as soon as the diagnosis is certain.

— Acceleration phase: 600 mg/d in a single dose.

— Blast phase: 600 mg/d as a single dose. [64]

Mechanisms of imatinib resistance :

Several mechanisms of resistance have been demonstrated: modification of the intracellular bioavailability of imatinib, over-expression of the MDR (multidrug resistance) gene, amplification of BCR-Abl, mutations in the kinase domain of Abl (>50 different mutations), BCR-Abl independent mechanisms. [40]

The criteria for resistance to imatinib are defined by the absence of hematological response at 3 months, the absence of cytogenetic response at 12 months or molecular relapse, i.e. an increase in the BCR-Abl transcript level in molecular biology of more than 2 logs on two consecutive tests carried out 1 month apart, or a persistent level of more than 10^2

The most frequently encountered mutations are located in the functional areas of the tyrosine kinase domain of Abl, within the BCR-Abl protein (exons 4 to 9 of *ABL1* corresponding to amino acids 240 to 500). Mutations affecting amino acids 250, 253 and 255 are located in the P loop (ATP phosphate binding site), T315I and F317L mutations in the hinge region between the N- and C-terminal lobes, mutations in 351, 355 and 359 upstream of the catalytic site and H396P/R substitutions in the A loop or activation loop [65].

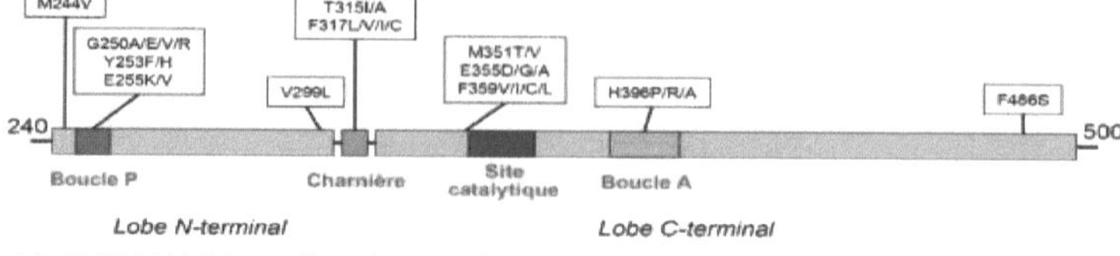

Figure 10: BCR/Abl kinase domain mutations [65].

4.2 Second-generation tyrosine kinase inhibitors

Three TKIs 2 (bosutinib, dasatinib, nilotinib) have been used in the treatment of chronic-phase CML intolerant or resistant to imatinib since 2005 in therapeutic trials, then as first-line therapy since 2008.

> **Dasatinib (Sprycel®, Bristol-Myers-Squibb)**

Is a TKI 325 times more potent *in vitro* than imatinib on non-mutated BCR-Abl.
It also inhibits Src family kinases. Study CA-180- 034
[23][66] demonstrated the value of its use in second-line treatment, and the Dasatinib *versus* Imatinib Study in Treatment-Naive CML Patients (DASISION) in 2010 [24][67] supported its use in first-line treatment, showing a better rate of complete cytogënëtic remission (*77%* versus 66% ; $p = 0.007$) at 12 months in patients receiving dasatinib 100 mg once daily versus imatinib 400 mg once daily indicated for the treatment of chronic, accelerated or blast phase CML in patients resistant to or intolerant of prior therapy including imatinib. [68,69]

> **Nilotinib (Tasigna®, Novartis)**

Is a structural analogue of imatinib, but its affinity for the ATP-binding site of the BCR-Abl protein is 50 times greater than that of imatinib *in vitro*, allowing *in vivo* hematological and cytological remission of patients who have failed treatment with imatinib. Its characteristics and chemical structure enable it to bypass Abl-kinase site mutations with the exception of the T315I mutation. [70]

Unlike imatinib and dasatinib, its pharmacokinetics require twice-daily administration. Its first-line use is based on the 2010 Evaluating Nilotinib Efficacy and Safety in Clinical Trials - Newly Diagnosed Patients (ENESTnd) trial, which showed a 12-month major molecular response (MMR) rate of 44% compared with 22% for imatinib ($p<0.001$). [71]

> **Bosutinib: BOSULIF® (in French)**

A "conditional authorisation" was granted on 27 March 2013 for Bosulif, which has demonstrated the ability to block the action of kinases in the SRC family and the oncoprotein
   Bcr-

Bosutinib is indicated for the treatment of CML in its three phases, when imatinib and other second-generation tyrosine kinase inhibitors are not considered appropriate treatments.

> In practice (**Appendix II**), if a patient is diagnosed with chronic-phase CML, treatment with TKIs should be initiated. Hydroxyurea may be used for cytoreduction pending formal diagnosis if leukocytosis exceeds 80 G/L.

The choice of TKI is open to debate. Studies have shown that dasatinib [67] and nilotinib , [71] but also, less unequivocally, the higher doses of imatinib [72]or the combination with interferon [73], provided better cytological, cytogënëtic and molecular response rates than imatinib at a dose of 400 mg/d.

Comparison by mëta-analysis of dasatinib and nilotinib shows their equivalence in terms of CCyR (complete cytogënëtic response) and MMR (major molecular response) [74]. However, the idea of preserving a second-line treatment in the event of failure of the first, i.e. first using imatinib at the conventional dose in order to keep open the possibility of treatment with a second-generation inhibitor in the event of a lack of response, has found supporters both for reasons of economy and treatment optimisation. The study needed to settle this question has yet to be undertaken.

> **Study of treatment response criteria and monitoring methods** (Appendix III)

Three levels of disease control can be defined in CML:

J Hematological response:

CHR (*complete hematological response)* is defined as the normalisation of the blood count and formula, (see platelet count, leucocytes, basophils and myeloma) and spleen size.

It must be achieved within 03 months of treatment to qualify as an optimal response. Blood counts are monitored every 02 weeks until CHR and then every 03 months.

J **Cytogenetic response :**

Is assessed by analysing at least 20 medullary metaphases.

It is called :

■ Minimum for the persistence of 66 to 95% of medullary metaphases containing the Philadelphia chromosome,

■ Minor for the persistence of 36% to 65% of positive metaphases,

■ Partial for the persistence of 1 to 35% of positive and complete metaphases (CCyR: complete cytogenetic response) in the absence of a Philadelphia chromosome on all the metaphases observed.

In order to achieve an optimal response, patients undergoing treatment must show at least a minimal cytogënëtic response at 03 months, a partial response at 06 months and a competitive response at 12 months.

■ If the response is only minor at six months, it's an **alert.**

■ The other cases, and the loss of CCyR, are treatment **failures** which should be the reason for a new course of treatment.

J **Molecular response :**

Among patients who have reached CCyR, two groups can still be distinguished prognostically, depending on whether or not the *BCR-ABL* fusion transcript remains detectable: MMR a done ëlë dë defined as an expression ratio of *BCR-Abl and a control gene less than or equal to 0.1% .* [75]

MMR (*major molecular response*) should be achieved within 18 months of treatment as part of an optimal response.

However, patients who do not achieve MMR are not considered to have failed treatment: this is an iK'cess alert requiring close follow-upë.

Loss of MMR, on the other hand, is considered a treatment failure. A so-called competitive molecular response (CMR) has ëlë dëfined as the indëtectabilitë of *BCR-Abl* in RT- PCR.

The recommendations of the European Leukemia Network (ELN) provide guidance for clinicians faced with alerts or failures. [76,77]

If treatment fails, a change of TKI must be immediately гёнHзё and an allograft may be proposed depending on the patient.

Table V: Dëfiиtion of initial responses to *imatinib* treatment according to the NLE. 2013. [35]

Moment	Pëacbon optimal	Alert	Failure
At the time of diagnosis	NA	High risk and/or ACA/Ph +.	NA
3 months	BCR–ABL< 10%, and/or Ph + <35%.	BCR–ABL >10%, and/or Ph+ 36 to	No RHC, and/or Ph+ > 95%.

		95%.	
6 months	BCR-ABL < 1%, and/or Ph+ 0	BCR-ABL 1% and 10%, and/or Ph+1 35	BCR-ABL > 10% and/or Ph+> 35%
12 months	BCR-ABL < 0.1	BCR-ABL 0.1 and 1	BCR-ABL > 1% and/or Ph+>0
At any time	BCR-ABL gene <0.1	ACA/Ph-(-7or-7q)	-Loss of RHC -Loss of RCYC -Loss conЛгтёе of the MMR* -Changes -ACA/PH+

- NA: Not applicable
- CHR: complete hematological response
- RCy: answer су1одёпёЬдие.
- RcyC: complete cytogenetic response.
- MMR: major molecular response
- ACA /Ph+: су1одёпёйдие additional anomaly whose Ph+ cells.
- ACA /Ph-: сугодёпёйдие additional anomaly whose Ph- cells.

Part II

The practice.

Reminder of the objectives of our study :

Main objective:

To study involution in CML by quantifying the BCR/Abl molecular transcript during the therapeutic phase.

Secondary objectives:

- Describe the patients' socio-demographic characteristics.
- Study of the kinetics of the BCR/Abl ratio during treatment.
- To study the therapeutic response to tyrosine kinase inhibitors (TKIs) in these patients.

1. Patients and methods

1. Description of the study

1.1. Type of study

This is a retrospective descriptive study of 30 cases who consulted the Matology Department of Tizi-Ouzou University Hospital over a period ranging from March 2010 to February 2018.

1.2. Study population

Our study included CML patients in whom BCR/Abl transcript quantification was performed before and after treatment.

1.3. Place of study

This study was carried out at the Hematology Department of CHU Nedir Mohamed in the wilaya of Tizi-Ouzou, particularly at the consultation unit.

1.4. Study period

This study was carried out over a period of 07 months, from November 2017 to May 2018.

2. Methodology

2.1. Information gathering

The data for our study were collected from the files of patients in the Hematology Department on the basis of an investigation form drawn up by ourselves (APPENDIX IV), including information concerning the patient's civil status (age, sex), clinical and para-clinical data (blood count formula, blood smear, liver and kidney function tests and molecular biology used to quantify the BCR/Abl molecular transcript by RT-PCR (APPENDIX IV).

2.2. Implementation phase

During the course of our study, we visited the hematology consultation and the archives at the Tizi-Ouzou University Hospital. Data was collected every Tuesday.

A sorting of the files was ël.ë efiectue, and we sëlectionnë patients with CML and in whom quantification of the BCR/Abl ratio was performed before and after treatment.

The data was collected from the files and reported on the survey forms.

During the study we subdivided our population into 3 groups of individuals according to their tolerance to ITKs.

- **1ᵉʳ group**: patients who progressed on imatinib 400mg.
- **2ᵉᵐᵉ group**: patients who progressed after failing imatinib 400mg with dose escalation to 600mg.
- **3ᵉᵐᵉ group**: patients who have failed imatinib 400 and 600mg using a 2ᵉᵐᵉ generation TKI.

2.3. Technique for quantifying the BCR/Abl molecular transcript :

The device used was the **GeneXpert**, whose quantification principle is based on RT-Q-PCR;

Principle :

Polymerase Chain Reaction (PCR) is an in vitro targeted replication technique. It is used to obtain large quantities of a specific nucleic acid fragment of defined length from a complex, low abundance sample.

Technical details :

Nucleic acid (transformed RNA or DNA), heat-resistant enzyme with buffer and magnesium chloride, ATGC bases and primers specific for the region to be amplified are placed in a tube. The tube is inserted into a thermal cycler and 35 cycles are run. Each cycle consists of 3 steps: Denaturation, Hybridization, Elongation

For molecular monitoring, we use quantitative PCR or real-time PCR or RQ PCR. In RQ-PCR we have two primers that bind to the complementary sëquence and between the two we add a probe marked by two fluorophores: one that is called a 5' reporter and the other a 3' quencher **(Appendix V).**

If the BCR- ABL transcript is present, the three PCR steps (denaturation, hybridization and elongation) are always performed.

Firstly, during elongation, the polymërase binds to the primer and begins to move along the strand. The probe is intact and the fluorescence intensity of the quencher is greater than that of the reporter.

Secondly: thanks to its exonuclease activity, it degrades the probe.

When the probe is cut, there is no longer any constraint on the reporter and the fluorescence of the reporter increases, so the fluorescence ratio is in favour of the reporter.

It is this increase in fluorescence that is detected and allows us to visualise the amplification.

(Appendix V)

Based on the Reporter-Quencher fluorescence ratio, we obtain a graphical representation of fluorescence intensity as a function of PCR cycles.

Obtaining quantification results :

The software will determine a threshold (which can be modified) as a function of the base fluorescence, and this threshold will be used to define Ct values. Ct are the PCR cycles at which the PCR is considered to be positive.

If a transcript range is used, a calibration curve can be plotted with the Concentrations as a function of quantity, thus determining the quantity of transcript (messenger RNA) present in the sample.

2.4.Statistical analysis

2.4.1. Definition of variables

We ëtudiës the following variables:

***J* Qualitative variables :**

- *Sex*: Male and Female
- *Reasons for consultation*: incidental findings, hyperleukocytosis, asthenia, bone pain, splenomegaly, weight loss, anaemia, visual blur.
- *Personal antecedents*: diabetes, hypertension, etc.
- *Clinical signs*: splenomegaly, asthenia, bone pain, anaemia, weight loss.

***J* Quantitative variables :**

- *Age*
- *White blood cell count*: in three ways:
- Less than 4000 elements/mm^3

- Between 4000 and 10000 elements/ mm^3
- More than 10000 elements/ mm^3 .
- **Haemoglobin level :**
- Less than 8 g/dl.
- Between 8 and 10 g/dl.
- Between 10 and 12 g/dl.
- Above 12 g/dl.
- **Platelet count :**
- Less than 120,000 elements/mm^3 .
- Between 120,000 and 500,000 elements/ mm^3 .
- More than 500,000 elements/ mm^3 .
- **Level of BCR/Abl molecular transcript :**
- CML: if the BCR/Abl ratio is greater than 10% at diagnosis.
- Early molecular response: if BCR/Abl ratio falls to less than 10%.
- Competing molecular response: if BCR/Abl ratio decreases to less than 1%.
- Major molecular response: if BCR/Abl ratio decreases to less than 0.1%.
- Deep molecular response: if BCR/Abl ratio decreases to less than 0.0032%.

2.4.2. Data entry and statistical tools used

The data was entered using the International Business Machine Statistical Package for Social Statistics version 20 "IBM SPSS Statistics 20" and Microsoft Excel 2016.

We carried out a descriptive analysis of the epidemiological and biological characteristics of the patients, as well as certain clinical and therapeutic data:

- For quantitative variables, we calculated the means with the standard deviation, and the percentage for qualitative variables.

- We used the classic parametric tests: **Wilcoxon test** to compare two means of a matched series, **Friedman test** to compare several means of a matched series.

- The significance level was set at a probability **p < 5% covering a confidence interval IC =95%.**

Results

1. Description of socio-demographic characteristics

1.1. Breakdown by age

The mean age of CML patients was ëlë 43.10 +/- 14.12 years with a minimum of 21 years and a maximum of 73 years.

1.2. Breakdown by age group

Occurrence ëlɯl: highest in subjects aged 30 to 50, with a frequency of 53.4% (Table VI) (Figure 11).

Table VI. Breakdown of patients by age group

Age group (years)	Workforce	Percentages	Cumulative percentages
[20-30[	6	20	20
[30-40[	8	26,7	46,7
[40-50[	8	26,7	73,4
[50-60[	4	13,3	86,7
[60-70[	3	10	96,7
[70-80[	1	3,3	100
Total	30	100	

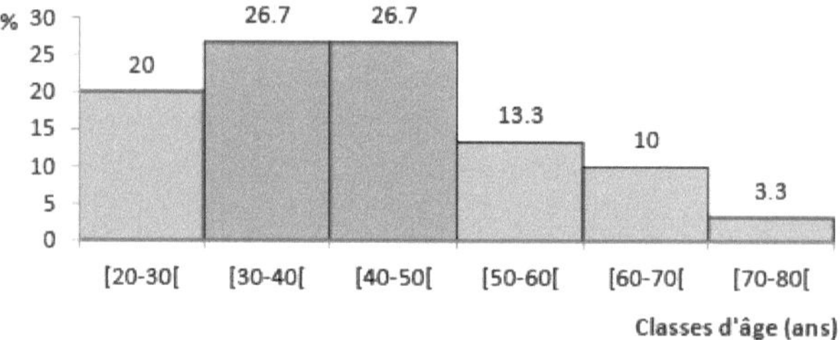

Figure 11. Rëpartition of CML patients according to age classes.

1.3. Breakdown by gender

In our study, the highest proportion of males was 56.7%, with a sex ratio of 1.3 (Table VII) (Figure 12).

Table VII. Distribution of patients by sex.

Gender	Workforce	Percentage
Male	17	56,7
Female	13	43,3
Total	30	100

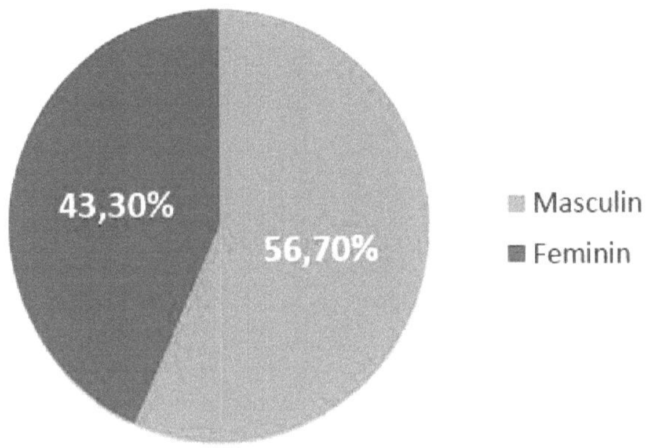

1.4.Breakdown by age and gender:

-The mean age of male patients was ëlë 43.43 +/- 13.24 years with a minimum of 28 years and a maximum of 70 years.

-The mean age of female patients was 42.69 +/- 15.75 years, with a minimum of 21 years and a maximum of 73 years.

2. Description of clinical and biological parameters.

2.1.Breakdown by circumstances of discovery:

In our sërie, 27 cases or (90%) of patients with CML had 1 hyperleukocytosis as a calling sign and 43.3% ëlë dë discovered incidentally. (Table VIII) (Figure 13)

Table VIII. Distribution of patients according to circumstances of discovery.

Reasons for consultation	Workforce	Percentages
Hyperleukocytosis	27	90
Fortuitous	13	43,3
Asthenia	10	33,3
Bone pain	5	16,7
Splenomegalia	4	13,3
Weight loss	2	6,7
Visual blur	2	6,7
Anemie	1	3,3

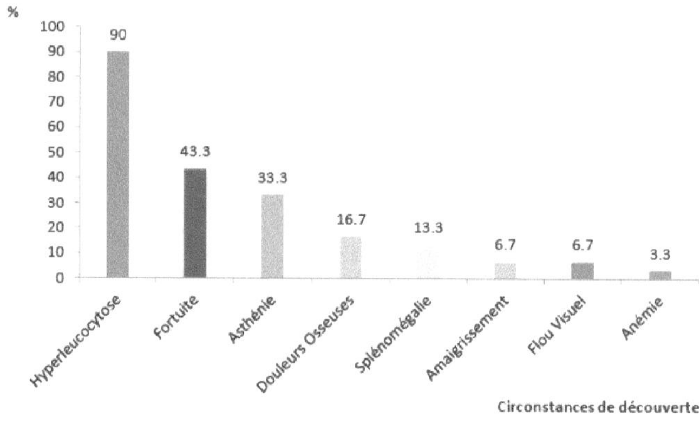

Figure 13. Breakdown of patients by reason for consultation.

2.2. Distribution of patients according to the presence or absence of personal antecedents :

In 63.3% of cases, no personal antëcëdent was encountered, whereas 36.7% of patients presented with: hypertension, diabëte, heart disease, surgery, etc. (Table IX) (Figure 14)

Table IX. Rëpartition of patients according to the presence or absence of personal antëcëdents.

Personal antdcddents	Workforce	Percentages
Present	11	36,7
Absent	19	63,3
Total	30	100

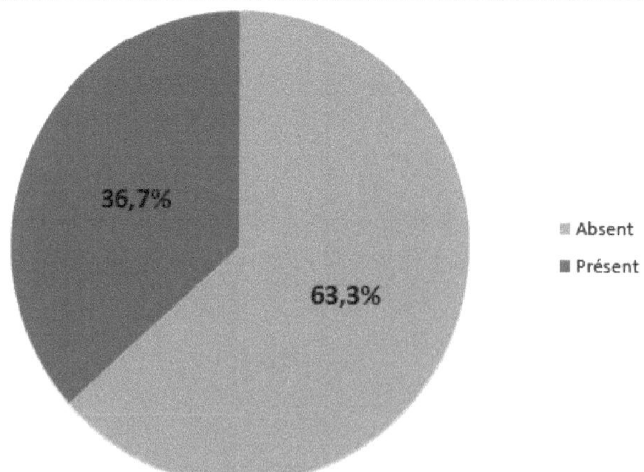

Figure 14. Distribution of patients according to the presence or absence of personal antëcëdents.

2.3. Clinical profile:

In our series, 66.6% of patients had splënomëgalia as a clinical sign of call, 23.30% had asthenia, and other clinical signs such as bone pain, anomia and weight loss were less

30

common (Table X) (Figure 15).

Table X. Distribution of patients according to clinical signs.

Clinical sign	Workforce	Percentages
Splenomegalia	20	66,6
Astienie	7	23,3
Bone pain	3	10
Anemie	3	10
Weight loss	2	6,7

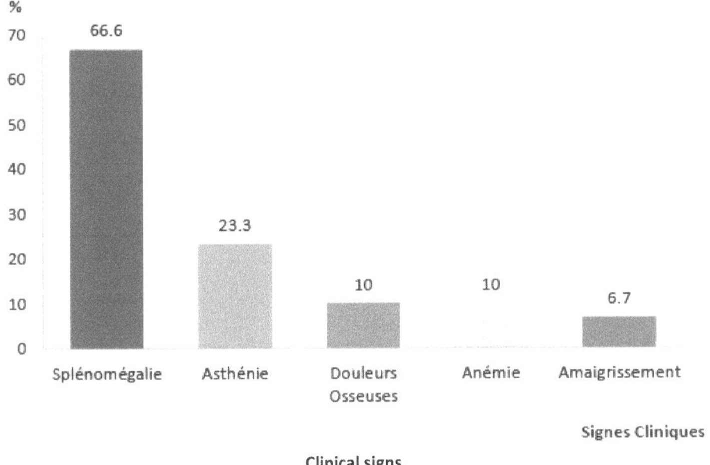

Figure 15. Distribution of patients according to clinical signs

2.4.Biological profile :

2.4.1. Blood count :

2.4.1.1.   White blood cells :

In our study, 100% of patients presented with hyperleukocytosis.

The mean leukocyte count was 236349.67± 313166.02 elets/mm^3 (236.34± 313.16 Giga/L) with a minimum of 25000 elets/mm^3 and a maximum of 1723000 elets/mm^3

2.4.1.2.   Haemoglobin:

A total of 36.7% had moderate anemia, 26.7% had mild anemia, 26.6% were normal and 10% had severe anemia (Table XI) (Figure 16).

Table XI. Distribution of patients according to hdmoglobin level at diagnosis.

Hemoglobin in g/dl	Workforce	Percentages	Cumulative percentages
[6-8[	3	10	10
[8-10[	11	36,7	46,7
[10-12[	8	26,7	73,4
[12-16[	8	26,6	100
Total	30	100	

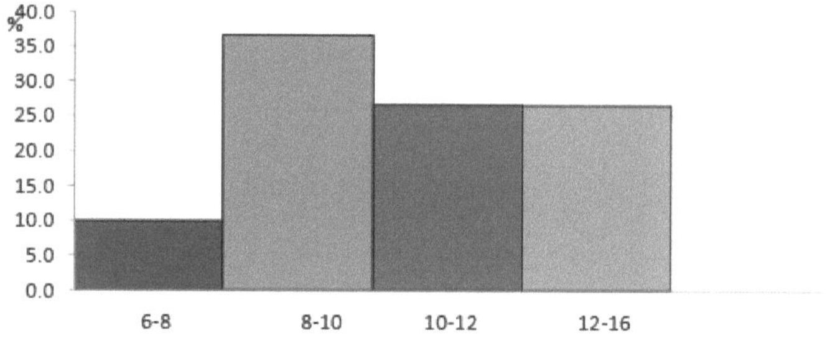

Figure 16. Distribution of patients according to hdmoglobin level at diagnosis.

2.4.1.3.   Platelets :

In our population, 66.7% of patients had a normal platelet count, 20% had a low platelet count and 20% had a high platelet count.

had thrombocytosis and 13.3% had tlirombopenia

(Table XII) (Figure 17).

Table XII. Distribution of patients according to platelet count in the diagnostic phase

Platelets (elets/mm)^3	Workforce	Percentages	Cumulative percentages
<120000	4	13,3	13,3
[120000-500000]	20	66,7	80
>500000	6	20	100
Total	30	100	

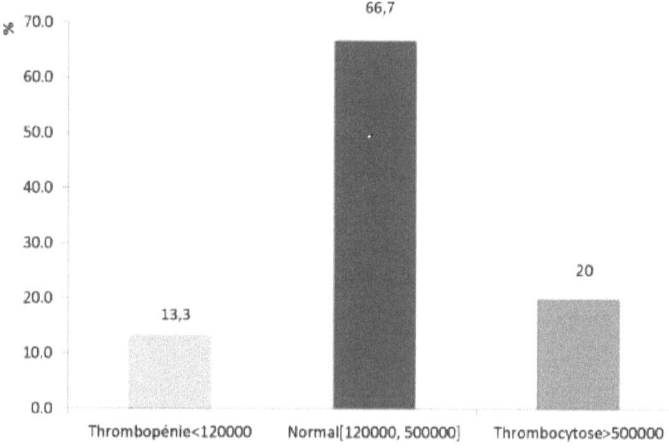

Figure 17. Distribution of patients according to platelet count in the diagnostic phase.

2.4.2. Blood smear balance:

All patients had a polynucldar count (PNN, PNE, PNB) ëlevës.

2.4.3. Molecular biology:

In our series, 56.6% of patients had a BCR ratio of 50 to 100%, 20% had a BCR ratio of 10 to 50% and 16.7% had a BCR ratio greater than 100%. (Table XIII) (Figure 18).

Table. XIII. Rëpartition of patients according to BCR/Abl ratio in the diagnostic phase.

BCR/Abl % rate	Workforce	Percentages	Cumulative percentages
0-10	2	6 ,7	6,7
10-50	6	20	26,7
50-100	17	56,6	83,3
>100	5	16,7	100
Total	30	100	

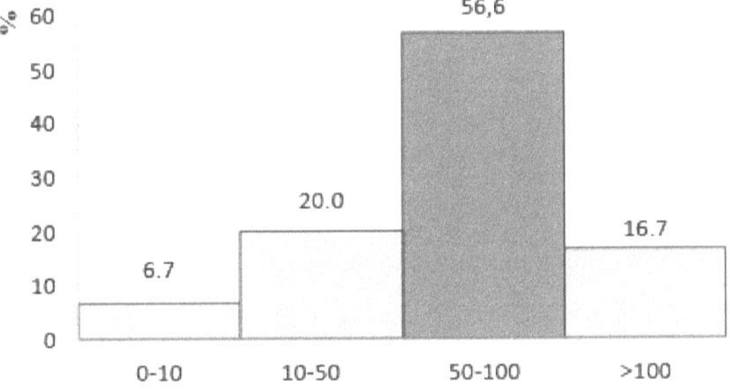

Figure 18. Distribution of CML patients according to BCR/Abl ratio in the diagnostic phase.

3. Prognostic assessment :

According to Sokal's classification; 36.7% of patients had a low risk, 33.3% had an intermëdiary risk and 30% had a high risk (Table XIV) (Figure 19).

Table XIV. Rëpartition of patients in our ëstudy according to Sockal's prognostic classification.

Prognostic classification	Workforce	Percentages	Cumulative percentages
High risk	9	30	30
Intermediate risk	10	33,3	66,3
Low risk	11	36,7	100
Total	30	100	

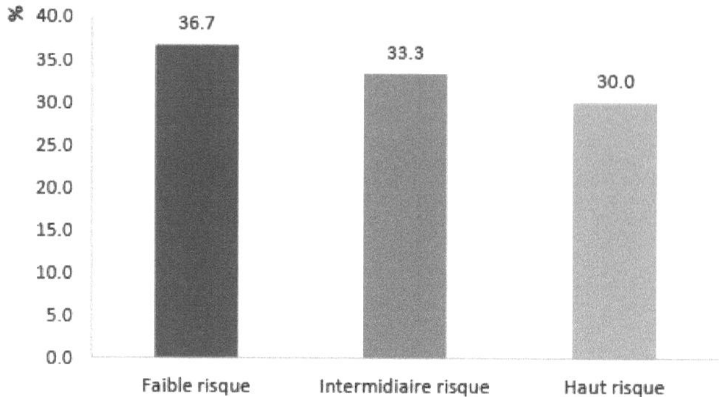

Figure 19. Rëpartition of patients according to Sockal's prognostic classification.

4. Evolution according to therapy :

4.1. Delay between diagnosis and treatment:

The mean time from diagnosis to administration of treatment in the patients in our study was 13.23 days +/- 10.37 with a minimum of 0 days and a maximum of 48 days.

4.2. Therapeutic monitoring according to the haemogram

4.2.1. Depending on the white blood cell count

Mean white blood cell counts tended to fall from 10134.67 ± 19837.85 elets/mm^3 at 3eme months after treatment to 6434.50 ± 3530.21 elets/mm^3 at 12eme months (Table XV) (Figure 20).

Table XV. Changes in white blood cell count during treatment

Processing time	N	Average white blood cell count (elets/mm)^3
3 Months	30	10134,67±19837,85
6 Months	30	7528,67±9668,10
12 Months	28	6434,50±3530,21

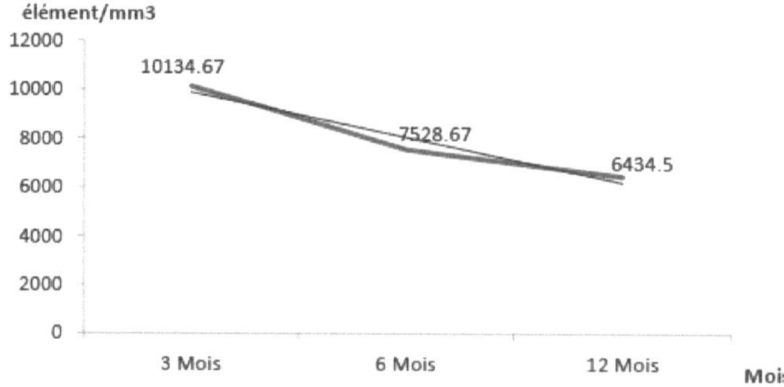

Figure 20: Changes in white blood cell count during treatment

4.2.2. Depending on the haemoglobin level :

Mean cnemoglobin values tended to increase from 11.62 ± 1.76 g/dl at 3eme months after treatment to 12.31 ± 1.66 g/dl at 12eme months (Table XVI) (Figure 21).

Table XVI. Changes in iemoglobin levels during treatment.

Treatment times	N	Mean iemoglobin (g /dl)
3 Months	30	11,62±1,76
6 Months	30	11,87±1,66
12 Months	28	12,31±1,66

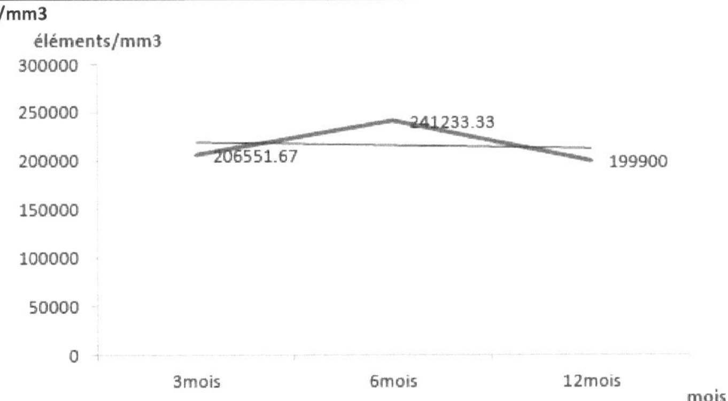

Figure 21. Changes in haemoglobin levels during treatment

4.2.3. Depending on the platelet count :

Mean platelet counts tended to stabilise during treatment. (Table XVII) (Figure 22).

Table XVII. Changes in platelet count during treatment.

Treatment times	N	Mean platelets ± ëstandard deviation
3 Months	30	206551,67±94740,46
6 Months	30	241233,33±194266,73
12 Months	28	199900±83458,20

elements/mm3

35

Figure 22. Changes in platelet count during treatment

4.3.Therapeutic monitoring based on molecular biology

4.3.1 Distribution of patients according to tolerance to treatment

- 1er group: patients who progressedë on imatinib 400mg.

- 2nd group: patients who had progressedë after failing imatinib 400mg followed by an increase in dose to 600mg.

- 3ёте group: patients who have failed 1 imatinib 400 and 600mg and for whom treatment with a2[^ʼ][e] generation TKI has ёlё administered.
(Table XVIII) (Figure 23)

In our series, 70% of patients are in group 1, 10% are in group 2 and 20% are in group 3.

Table XVIII. Distribution of patients according to tolerance to treatment.

The groups	Workforce	Percentages	Cumulative percentages
Group 1	21	70	70
Group 2	3	10	80
Group 3	6	20	100
Total	30	100	

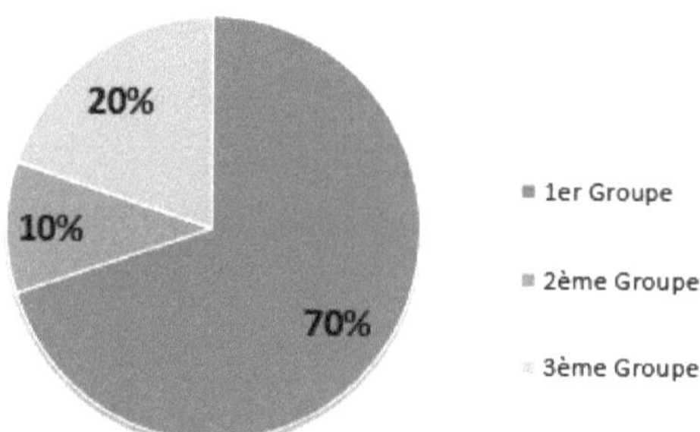

Figure 23. Distribution of patients according to treatment tolerance.

4.3.2. Monitoring changes in the BCR/Abl molecular transcript ratio

4.3.2.1. Monitoring of the BCR/Abl molecular transcript ratio in patients in group 1.

Mean values for the BCR/Abl molecular transcript ratio tended to fall from 1.82±2.32% at 3[eme] months after treatment to 0.12±0.17% at 34[eme] months (Table XIX) (Figure 24).

Table XIX. Change in BCR/Abl ratio during treatment in group 1 patients.

Treatment timesN	Mean BCR /Abl ratio ± standard deviation
6 Months15	1,82±2,32
12 Months6	0,15±0,15
24 Months8	0,08±0,14
34 Months4	0,12±0,17

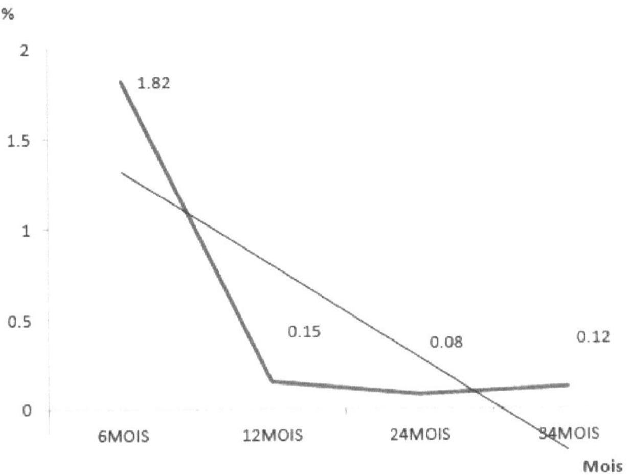

Figure 24. Changes in BCR/Abl levels during treatment in group 1 patients.

4.3.2.2. Monitoring of the evolution of the BCR/Abl molecular transcript ratio in patients in group 2.

Mean values for the BCR/Abl molecular transcript ratio tended to fall from 2.7±2.20% at 6eme months after treatment to 2.15±1.76% at 18eme months (Table XX) (Figure 25).

Table XX. Change in BCR/Abl ratio during treatment in group 2.

Treatment times	N	Mean BCR /Abl ratio ± standard deviation
6 Months	3	2,7±2,20
12 Months	2	1,05±0,49
18 Months	2	2,15±1,76

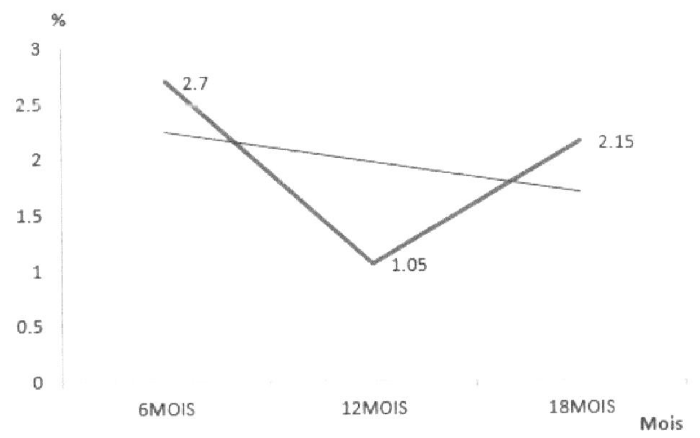

Figure 25. Change in BCR/Abl ratio during treatment in patients in group 2.

4.3.2.3. The evolution of the BCR/Abl molecular transcript ratio was monitored in patients in group 3.

Mean values for the BCR/Abl molecular transcript ratio tended to fall from 21% at 6eme

months after treatment to 0.13±0.10% at 34eme months (Table XXI) (Figure 26).

Tableau XXI. Change in BCR/Abl ratio during treatment in group 3.

Treatment time	N	MeanBCR /Abl ratio ± ëstandard deviation
6 Months	1	21
12 Months	3	25,25±18,46
18 Months	3	16,08±27,64
24 Months	3	12,6±18,76
34 Months	3	0,13±0,10

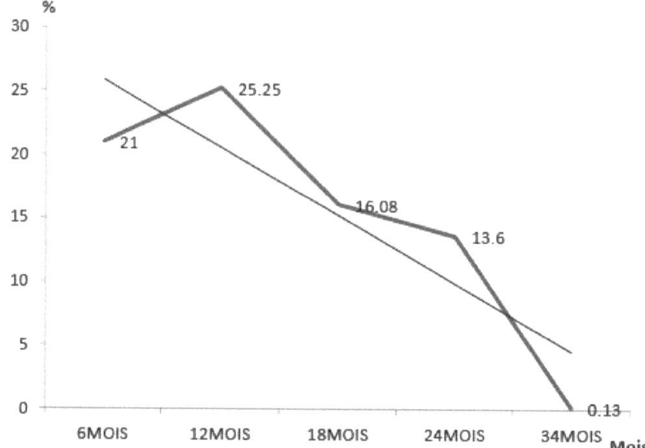

Figure 26. Change in BCR/Abl ratio during treatment in group 3 patients.

5. Changes in various biological parameters during the therapeutic phase

- The mean WBC was 10134.67±19837.85 at 3eme months, with no statistically significant difference from the means at 6eme and 12eme months, which were 10134.67±19837.85 and 6434.5±3530.21 respectively (p= 0.13).

- The mean Hb level was 11.62±1.76 at 3eme months with no statistically significant difference from the means at 6eme and 12eme which were 11.87±1.66 and 12.31±1.66 respectively (p=0.26).

- The average platelet count was 206551.67±9740.46 at 3eme months, with no statistically significant difference from the averages at 6eme and 12eme , which were 241233.33±194266.73 and 199900±83458.20 respectively (p=0.62).

- The mean BCR/Abl ratio before treatment was 108.03±158.69 higher than that after treatment, which was 0.31±0.69 with a statistically significant difference (p<10^{-4}) (Table XXII).

Tableau XXII. Rëpartition of patients according to Involution of different biological parameters during the ^therapeutic phase.

Përiode of dosage	N	Mean ± ëstandard deviation	P
GB	28		
3 months		10134,67±19837,85	DNS
6 months		7528,67±9668,10	P=0,13
12 months		6434,5±3530,21	

Hb	28		
3 months		11,62±1,76	
6 months		11,87±1,66	DNS
12 months		12,31±1,66	p=0,26
BCR/Abl ratio	23		
Before treatment		108,03±158,69	DS
After treatment		0,31±0,69	$p<10^{-4}$

<h1>Discussion</h1>

1. Limits of the study

The data analysed were collected retrospectively from medical records and files, which made it difficult to use them.

The size of the sample was a ë1.ë limiting factor in the analysis of the data; in fact, the number of CML patients whose BCR/Abl molecular transcript level was quantified before and after treatment is notably low, i.e. 30 cases since 2012. An average of 5 patients per year.

In addition, some files were not fully completed, and we were faced with a lack of patient follow-up data and a loss of files due to poor archiving conditions.

2. Study biases

As with any research study, some biases were introduced into our work:

- A selection bias, as several patients benefited from quantification of the BCR/Abl ratio either before or after treatment only.
- Information bias: during data collection, we provided a certain amount of information that was not systematically available in the files.
- A memory bias linked to an omission on the part of the doctor and/or patient to report certain facts or information on the file.
- A measurement bias that is linked to errors that may be caused by the automatic machines, the reading of the cards, the karyotype, etc.
- A prevarication bias: patients may give erroneous information about their state of health when questioned by the doctor.

3. Discussion of the results and comparison with national and international studies:

Our study enabled us to demonstrate that there is a relationship between the quantification of the BCR/Abl molecular transcript and the therapeutic response, which progressively improved, leading us to observe an MMR, an indication of the patients' healing pathway.

Our results were as follows:

The study population comprised adult patients with a mean age of 43.10 +/- 14.12 years, with a minimum of 21 years and a maximum of 73 years. A high frequency of CML cases was observed in the 30-50 age group. These data are consistent with those of the Algerian series [37], and the two Moroccan series [43,78], unlike the French series [79] whose mean age was 63 years and whose most affected age group was 60 to 80 years; this difference could be explained by the young age of the Algerian and Moroccan populations.

Our series is predominantly male, with a sex ratio of 1.3, which is in line with the literature. [37,43, 79]

In our series, 90% of patients with CML had hyperleukocytosis as a sign of call because we were talking about a myeloproliferative syndrome in which the abnormal multiplication of bone marrow cells is predominantly polynuclear;

Almost 43.3% of patients discovered CML incidentally, which may be explained by the fact that CML is a latent disease with a long period of clinical expression.

Clinically, all the patients in our study presented a certain number of clinical signs, including splenomegaly, which was found in the majority of cases (66.6%). Similar results have been reported in the literature. [43, 44,80]

Biologically, we found that all patients had hyperleukocytosis, so their blood smears showed a considerable increase in polynuclear cell counts. The hemoglobin level also fell (< 12 g/dl), causing anaemia in 73.4% of patients. This could be due to excessive proliferation of leukemia cells, which disrupts erythropoiesis.

At diagnosis, molecular biology showed that 56.6% of patients had a BCR/Abl ratio between 50 and 100%, and 16.7% had a BCR/Abl ratio greater than 100%. These high figures resulted in a mean time from diagnosis to treatment of 13.23 +/- 10.37 days, allowing early therapeutic follow-up of patients. These data are consistent with those in the literature [2].

According to Sokal's prognostic classification, we found a predominance of low risk. This result is discordant with that of the study [3] where we found a predominance of high risk; this could be due to the early diagnosis of CML in the patients in our population.

During the management of the patients, therapeutic follow-up was established based on the haemogram and molecular biology, enabling a better assessment of the therapeutic response.

However, mean white blood cell counts tended to fall from 10134.67 ± 19837.85 at 3eme months after treatment to 6434.50 ± 3530.21 elements/mm^3 at 12eme months, which is a normal level. However, the results of the literature [3] showed considerable leukopenia, which could be due to the side effects of the TKI treatment taken by the patients in the study [3].

After subdivision of the population into 3 cohorts according to tolerance to treatment, it turned out that the first group contained 70% of patients who had MMR on imatinib 400 mg, the second group included 10% of patients who did not progress on imatinib 400 mg and for whom the doctor increased the dose to 600 mg, and finally the third group included 20% of patients who had failed on imatinib 400 and 600 mg. These patients were substituted with a second-generation TKI. These results are consistent with the literature [3].

All patients had an assessment of their response to imatinib; however, they had a considerable reduction in the BCR/Abl level after 12 months, and then the patients in group 2 experienced an increase in the BCR/Abl level, which enabled us to establish a failure of imatinib 400 mg, so the dose had to be increased to 600 mg, so we noticed a progression.

And for patients in group 3, we observed a progression as the BCR/Abl level fell considerably in association with second-generation TKIs.

The mean BCR/Abl ratio before treatment was ëlë 108.03 ± 158.69 higher than that after treatment, which was ëlë 0.31 ± 0.69 with a significant difference (p<10-4). These results are consistent with the literature [81,82].

Similarly, a Tunisian study carried out along these lines, rëalisëed by Menif et al in 2009 [83] showed that patients who had been monitored by BCR/Abl quantification had all progressed after 12 months. Detection of minute amounts of this level after 24 months showed that 96% of patients ëwere on their way to gi^rison. [84]

Finally, we foundë discrepancies between our results and some of the literature; this implies the need for further studies that can be verified by other research projects.

Conclusion and recommendations

We carried out a retrospective and descriptive study on the quantification of the BCR/ABL molecular transcript at diagnosis and in the follow-up of patients with CML treated with TKIs.

Our study involved 30 patients treated in the haematology department of Tizi Ouzou University Hospital, at the consultation unit. Molecular follow-up was carried out for a median period of 24 months (3-34) after the start of treatment.

Depending on the population studied, we can conclude that molecular monitoring of CML reveals a number of particularities, the main ones being :

- An average age of 43.10 +/- 14.12 years, with a minimum of 21 and a maximum of 73.
- Males accounted for the highest proportion at 56.7%, with a sex ratio of 1.3.
- 66.6% of patients had spldnomdalgia as a clinical sign.
- 56.6% of patients were diagnosed with a BCR:Abl ratio of 50 to 100%.
- According to Sokal's prognostic classification, we found a predominance of low risk.
- Molecular follow-up showed that 70% of patients achieved MMR with imatinib 400 mg.
- 20% of patients who had failed imatinib 400 and 600 mg were substituted with a second-generation TKI (nilotinib) and 100% MMR was observed
- Quantification of the BCR/Abl ratio showed that 96% of patients on imatinib 400mg were on the road to recovery.

Optimising treatment, adjusting it and using the various TKIs available therefore requires biomolecular monitoring of BCR/Abl transcripts from diagnosis onwards, in order to assess residual disease. This biological approach is not only essential for confirming the diagnosis of CML, but also for ensuring therapeutic follow-up and efficacy.

At the end of our study, we can make the following suggestions:

- To continue this work over a longer period in order to obtain results enabling long-term clinical follow-up, which is currently essential to determine the impact of molecular monitoring on patient outcome,

- Strengthening the technical capacity of laboratories for early and accurate diagnosis:

o Implement conventional diagnostic cytogënëtic techniques to search for the Ph chromosome

o Systëmatisation of molecular biology to search for and quantify BCR/ABL transcripts by RQ-PCR, in order to refine monitoring, assess the efficacy of TKI treatment and measure a major molecular response.

References

1. R. Mertelsmann, M. Engelhardt, D. P. Berger.Precis d'liematologie et d'oncologie. Paris Heidelberg New York 2010: 978-2-287-993,

2. Sandhya Sreenivasan Tantuan, Hanri du Plessis, Monique Stemmet1, Christopher D. Viljoen, Quantification of BCR-ABL1 on the GeneXpert: From diagnostics to research Department of Hematology and Cell Biology, University of the Free State, Bloemfontein, South Africa

3. N. MESSAOUDI. Leucëmie myeloide chronique chez l'adulte, iaculte de medecine, Bedjaya .2016

4. Piller, G. J. "Leukaemia, a brief historical review from ancient times to 1950." British Journal of Haematology.(2001).

5. Tefferi, A. "The history of myeloproliferative disorders: before and after Dameshek." (2008).

6. Nowell, P. C., Hungerford, D.A. "Chromosome Studies on Normal and Leukemic Human Leukocytes." JNCI J Natl Cancer Inst, (1960).

7. Rowley, J. D. "A New Consistent Chromosomal Abnormality in Chronic Myelogenous Leukaemia identified by Quinacrine Fluorescence and Giemsa Staining." Nature 243, (1973): 290 - 293.

8. MOZZICONACCI, Doctor Marie-Joelle. History of Chronic Myëloid Leukëmia (CML), 2015. http://www.lmc-france.fr/la-lmc/qu-est-ce-que-la-lmc/historique-de-la-lmc/ accessed 20 04 2016.

9. http://www.fnclcc.fr, FNCLCC (Federation nationale des centres de lutte contre.

10. Sebahoun G. Clinical and biological lenmitology. Arnette groupe liaisons SA.

11. Bergerat JP, Dufour P, Oberling F. Oncohematology. Heures de France, Toiry.

12. Chronic Myelogenous Leukemia and Related Disorders:Overview Williams Haematology 2007>PartIX.Malignant Diseases>Chapter88

13. T. Leguay, F.-X. Mahon *Chronic myelogenous leukaemia (2005)

14. Thierry Lavabre-Bertrand, Eric Jourdan, Jean Paul Bureau, Pierre Blanc. Liver and myeloproliferative disorders. Gastroenterol Clin Biol 2002; 26: 136145.

15. Redhouane, Pr Ahmed Nacer.revue algerienne d'hematologe, leucemie myeloide chronique: aspect epidemiologique . 2010.

16. R. Mertelsemenn, M. Engelhardt, D.P. Berger. Precis d'hematologie et d'oncologie. Springer-Verlag France, Paris 2011.

17. Deininger MW, Bose S, Gora-Tybor J, Yan XH, Goldman JM, Melo JV. Selective induction of leukemia-associated fusion genes by high-dose ionizing radiation. Cancer Res 1998; 58: 421-5.

18. G. Dine,, Y. Rehn, S. Brahimi, N. Ali Ammar, B. Gaillard,Y. Bocq, G. Fumagalli. *Residual disease in chronic myeloid leukemia,*Immunoanalysis and specialised biology (2013).

19. de Klein A, van Kessel AG, Grosveld G, Bartram CR, Hagemeijer A, Bootsma D, et al. A cellular oncogene is translocated to the Philadelphia chromosome in chronic myelocytic leukaemia. *Nature* 1982;300:765-7.

20. Thijsen S, Schuurhuis G, van Oostveen J, Ossenkoppele G. Chronic myeloid leukemia from basics to bedside. *Leukemia* 1999;13:1646-74.

21. Goldman JM, Melo JV. Chronic myeloid leukemia-advances in biology and new

approaches to treatment. *N Engl J Med* 2003;349:1451-64.

22. Pane F, Frigeri F, Sindona M, Luciano L, Ferrara F, Cimino R, et al. Neutrophilic-chronic myeloid leukemia: a distinct disease with a specific molecular marker (BCR/ABL with C3/A2 junction). *Blood* 1996;88:2410-4.

23. Thierry Lavabre-Bertrand, Eric Jourdan, Jean Paul Bureau, Pierre Blanc. Liver and myeloproliferative syndromes. Gastroenterol Clin Biol 2002; 26: 136-145.

24. Ren R. Mechanisms of BCR-ABL in the pathologenes of chronic myelogenous leukemia. Nat Rev Cancer 2005; 5: 172-83.

25. Jamieson CH, Ailles LE, Dylla SJ, Muijtjens M, Jones C, Zehnder JL, et al.Granulocyte-macrophage progenitors as candidate leukemic stem cells in blast-crisis CML. N Engl J Med 2004; 351: 657-67.

26. -M. Maigre, JL. Harrousseau. Leucemie myeloide chronique : acquisitions recentes. Le concours medical;1990 :112-19.

27. Gambacorti-Passerini C, Kantarjian HM, Baccarani M. Activity and tolerance ofbosutinib in patients with AP and BP CLM and Ph+ ALL. J Clin Oncol. 2008;

28. Sebahoun G. Hematologie clinique et biologique. Arnette groupe liaisons SA,Rueil-Malmaison 2005; 578 pages.

29. Treuil P. Chronic myeloid leukemia and its treatment with imatinib. Act Pharm 2008; 474: 25-30.

30. T. Leguay, F.-X Mahon. Chronic myeloid leukemia. EMCHematologie2 (2005) 187 205.

31. Sebahoun G. Clinical and biological lenmitology. Arnette groupe liaisons SA, Rueil-Malmaison 2005; 578 pages.

32. Treuil P. Chronic myeloid leukemia and its treatment with imatinib. Act Pharm 2008; 474: 25-30.

33. Thiebaud, M. Dubreuil. Clinical study of chronic myeloid leukaemia. EMC 13011 B-7, 1986.

34. Iansen JA, Gooley TA, Martin PJ, Appelbaum F, Chauncey TR, Clift RA, et al. Bone marrow transplants from unrelated donors for patients with chronic myeloid leukemia.NEnglJMed1998;338:962-8

35. European Leukemia Net recommendations for the management of chronic myeloid leukemia, 2013 version. (Baccarani, M et al: Blood, 2013; Vol. 122: 872-84).

36. Iuntly BJ, Bench A, Green AR. Double jeopardy from a single translocation: deletions of the derivative chromosome 9 in chronic myeloid leukemia. Blood 2003; 102: 1160-8.

37. Iamladji Rose Marie, Belhani Meriem, Ardjoun Fatma Zohra, Abad Mohand Tayeb, Touhami Iadj, Ait Ali Iocine, et al. Leucemie myeloide chronique, Aspects epidemiologique, diagnostique et therapeutique en Algerie, Revue Algerienne d'Hematologie N° 3. September 2010, p. 1-42.

38. Chrystele Bilhou-Nabera, Carole Barin, Alain Bernheim, Nicole Dastugue, Virginie Eclache, Claude Leonard,. Recommendations for the cytogenetic management of chronic myeloid leukemia (CML) established by the Groupe Frangais de Cytogenetique Iematologique (GFCI). Pathologie Biologie 52 (2004) 238 240.

39. Dominique Bories, Agnes Devergie, Martine Gardembas-Pain, Mathieu Kuentz, Laurence Legros, Francois- Guilhot. Therapeutic strategies and recommendations for the management of patients with chronic myeloid leukaemia. Iematologie. Volume 9, Number 6, 497-512, November-December 2003, Revue.

40. Tome 2, I leimitologie clinique, La leucëmie myeloide chronique R. LACROIX, F. SABATIER, F. DIGNAT-GEORGE et J. SAMPOL Laboratoire d'immunologie et d'hematologie, UFR de pharmacie, Aix-Marseille Universite.

41. Branford S, lughes T, Rudzki Z, et al. Monitoring chronic myeloid leukaemia therapy by real-time quantitative PCR in blood is a reliable alternative to bone marrow cytogenetics Br J laematol 2003 ; 107 : 587-99.

42. Virginie Eclache, Franooise Lejeune. Chromosome detection Philadelphia in patients with chronic myeloid leukemia, the respective roles of cytogenetics, fluorescence in situ hybridization and molecular analysis by RT-PCR. Revue Frangaise des Laboratoires, January 2002, N°339 **43.** M.l Guerraoui . Leucemie myeloide chronique : aspects évolutifs et therapeutiques. These en medecine. Faculte de MED V de Rabat 1997; 225.

44. AGlARBI Fatima-Zahra. Chronic myeloid leukaemia: diagnostic and therapeutic advances. Faculte de medecine de Fes 2008 86-08

45. Speck B, Bortin MM, Champlin R, Goldman JM, lerzig Rl, McGlave PB, et al. Allogeneic bone-marrow transplantation for chronic myelogenous leukaemia. *Lancet* 1984;**1**: 665-8.

46. Course on myeloproliferative disorders at the University of Rennes 1 in November 2006

47. Course on myeloproliferative disorders at the University of Rennes 1 in November 2006

48. Sokal JE, Cox EB, Baccarani M, *et al.* Prognostic discrimination in "good-risk" chronic granulocytic leukemia. *Blood* 1984; 63: 789-99.

49. lasford J, Pfirrmann M, lehlmann R, *et al.* A new prognosticscore for survival of patients with chronic myeloid leukemia treated with interferon alfa. Writing Committee for the Collaborative CML Prognostic Factors Project Group. *J Natl Cancer Inst* 1998; 90: 8508.

50. Hasford J, Baccarani M, Hoffmann V, *et al.* Predicting complete cytogenetic response and subsequent progression-free survival in 2060 patients with CML on imatinib treatment: the EUTOS score. *Blood* 2011; 118: 686-92.

51. Druker BJ, Talpaz M, Resta DJ, *et al.* Efficacy and safety of a specific inhibitor of the BCR-ABL tyrosine kinase in chronic myeloid leukemia. *N Engl J Med* 2001; 344: 1031-7.

52. Hehlmann R, Heimpel H, Hasford J, Kolb HJ, Pralle H, Hossfeld DK, et al.Randomized comparison of interferon-alpha with busulfan and hydroxyurea in chronic myelogenous leukemia. The German CML Study Group. Blood1994; 84:4064-77.

53. Ph. DOROSZ. Gide pratique des mëdicaments. 22nd edition. 2002

54. P. Rousselot, H. Rochant, A.G. Turhan, A. Bernheim, D. Bories, C. Recher, J. Bпёге, A. Najman, L. Sutton, A. Buzyn, A. Devergie. Update on chronic тyё^Mc leukëmia. Mëdecine tlK'rapeutique. Volume 6, Numëro 2, 129-40, Fëvrier 2000.

55. M. Benakli, RM. Hamladji, R. Ahmed-nacer. Hëmatopoiëtic stem cell allograft conditioning айёпиё. Sociëtë algerienne d'liematologie et de transfusion sanguine. Jan 26, 2013.

56. Guilhot F. Diagnosis and treatment of malignant hëmopathies involving a bcr-abl rearrangement I kmatologie 1995; 1: 133-144.

57. Labussiëre H, Hayette S, Tigaud I, Michallet M, Nicolini FE. The treatment of chronic myëloid leukëmia in 2007. Bull Cancer 2007; 94: 863-869.

58. Guilhot F, Roy L, Guilhot J, Millot F. Interferon therapy in chronic myelogenous leukemia. Hematol Oncol Clin N Am 2004; 18: 584-603.

59. Lacotte-Thierry L, Guilhot F. Interfëron and hëmatology. Rev Med Interne 2002; 23:

481-488.

1.1. Druker BJ, Tamura S, Buchdunger E, *et al.* Effects of a selective inhibitor of the Abl tyrosine kinase on the growth of Bcr-Abl positive cells. *Nat Med* 1996; 2: 561-6.

61. M.Tulliez. A new treatment for chronic myeloid leucëmia: l'imatinib (glivec*). Revue frangaise des laboratoires ; dëcembre 2003 ; n°358.

62. Bardin C, Tafzi N, Decleves X, Huet E, Chast F. Pharmacokinetics of tyrosine kinase inhibitors in chronic myeloid leukemia. Rev Francoph Lab 2007; 395: 31-35.

63. Peng B, Hayes M, Resta D, Racine-Poon A, Drucker BJ, Talpaz M, et al. Pharmacokinetics and pharmacodynamics of imatinib in a phase I trial with chronic myeloid leukemia patients. J Clin Oncol 2004; 22: 935-942.

64. Labussiere H, Hayette S, Tigaud I, Michallet M, Nicolini FE. The treatment of chronic myeloid leucëmia in 2007. Bull Cancer 2007; 94: 863-869.

65. Jean-Claude Chomela,* Biologie moleculaire de la leucemie myeloide Chronique / REVUE FRANCOPHONE DES LABORATOIRES - MAI 2017 -

1.1. Shah NP, Cortes JE, Schiffer CA, *et al.* Five-year follow-up of patients with imatinib-resistant or -intolerant chronic-phase chronic myeloid leukemia (CML-CP) receiving dasatinib. *J Clin Oncol* 2011; 29(Suppl. 1): abstract 6512.

67. Kantarjian H, Shah NP, Hochhaus A, *et al.* Dasatinib *versus* imatinib in newly diagnosed chronic-phase chronic myeloid leukemia. *N Engl J Med* 2010; 362: 2260-70.

68. Buxeraud J, Skrzypek A. Sprycel® - dasatinib. Act pharm 2008; 471.

69. Therapeutic innovations outside the ATU. Dossier dispensation. Act pharm hospitalieres 2007; 12.

70. Rosti G. A phase II study of nilotinib administered to imatinib resistant and intolerant patients with chronic myelogenous leukemia in chronic phase, ASCO Annual meeting (2007) abstract 7007.

71. Saglio G, Kim DW, Issaragrisil S, *et al.* Nilotinib *versus* imatinib for newly diagnosed chronic myeloid leukemia. *N Engl J Med* 2010; 362: 2251-9.

72. Alattar M, Kantarjian H, Jabbour E, *et al.* Clinical significance of complete cytogenetic response (CCyR) and major molecular response (MMR) achieved with different treatment modalities used as frontline therapy in chronic myeloid leukemia (CML) chronic phase (CP) [abstract]. *Blood* 2011; 118: abstract 745 (ASH Annual Meeting Abstracts).

73. Simonsson B, Gedde-Dahl T, Markevarn B, *et al.* Combination of pegylated IFN-alpha2b with imatinib increases molecular response rates in patients with low- or intermediate-risk chronic myeloid leukemia. *Blood* 2011 ; 118 : 3228-35.

74. Mealing S, Barcena L, Hawkins N, *et al.* The relative efficacy of imatinib, dasatinib and nilotinib for newly diagnosed chronic myeloid leukemia: a systematic review and network meta-analysis. *Exp Hematol Oncol* 2013; 2: 5.

75. Hughes T, Deininger M, Hochhaus A, *et al.* Monitoring CML patients responding to treatment with tyrosine kinase inhibitors: review and recommendations for harmonizing current methodology for detecting BCR-ABL transcripts and kinase domain mutations and for expressing results. *Blood* 2006; 108: 28-37.

76. Baccarani M, Pileri S, Steegmann JL, *et al.* Chronic myeloid leukemia: ESMO clinical practice guidelines for diagnosis, treatment and follow-up. *Ann Oncol* 2012; 23: vii72-7.

77. Baccarani M, Cortes J, Pane F, *et al.* Chronic myeloid leukemia: an update of concepts and management recommendations of European LeukemiaNet. *J Clin Oncol* 2009; 27: 6041 51.

78. Ms EL MOUHDI GHIZLAN, THE CINICAL AND CYTOGENETIC ASPECTS OF CHRONIC MYLOID LEUCEMIA, These питёго 186/15, 2015.

79. Maynadië M., Le Guyader-Peyrou S., Delafosse P., Mounier M., Collignon A., Troussard X., Monnereau A. Chronic myeloid leukëmia. Revue : Estimation nationale de 1'incidencedes cancers en France entre 1980 et 2012 (Etude a partir des registres des cancers du reseau Francim - Partie 2 - I E'mo|pitliies malignes), 2013, vol. 2, p.68-71.

80. A.Benabdeljelil .un visage de LMC au Maroc. These en mëdecine a la facu№ de rabat 1980 n°38.

81. Kantarjian HM, Talpaz M, Cortes J, et al. Quantitative polymerase chain reaction monitoring of bcr-abl during therapy with imatinib mesylate(STI 571) in chronic phase chronic myelogenous leukaemia. Clin cancer
Reseach 2003;9:160-6.

82. Merx K, Muller MC, Kreil S, et al. Early m RNA transcript levels predict cytogenetic response in chronic phase CML patients treated with imatinib after failure of interferon alpha. Leukemia 2002;16:1579-83.

83. S. Menif ,, S. Zarrouki , R. Jeddi , N. ben Alaya , Z. BelHadj Ali , H. Ben Abid ,
Quantitative detection of bcr-abl transcripts in chronic myeloid leukemia, Laboratoire d'liematologie moleculaire et cellulaire, institut Pasteur de Tunis, Tunis, Tunisia , Service d'liematologie, hopital Aziza-Othmana, Tunis, Tunisia , Service d'hematologie, hopital Farhat-Hached-Sousse, Tunis, Tunisia
Service c'hematology, hopital Hadi-Chacker Sfax, Tunis, Tunisia
Received 22 December 2006; accepted 14 December 2007 Available online 2 April 2008

84. Iacobucci I, Saglio G, Rosti G, et al. Achieving a major molecular response at the time of a complete cytogenetic response predicts a better duration of CCR in imatinib treated chronic myeloid leukemia patients. Clin cancer Research 2006.

APPENDIX I. Cell signalling pathways. The Bcr-Abl protein activates different signalling signalling pathways. For simplicity, the main ones are shown here. However, a large number of identified as being directly or indirectly phosphorylated by the kinase activity of Bcr-Abl. phosphorylated by the kinase activity of Bcr-Abl.

Bcr-Abl protein

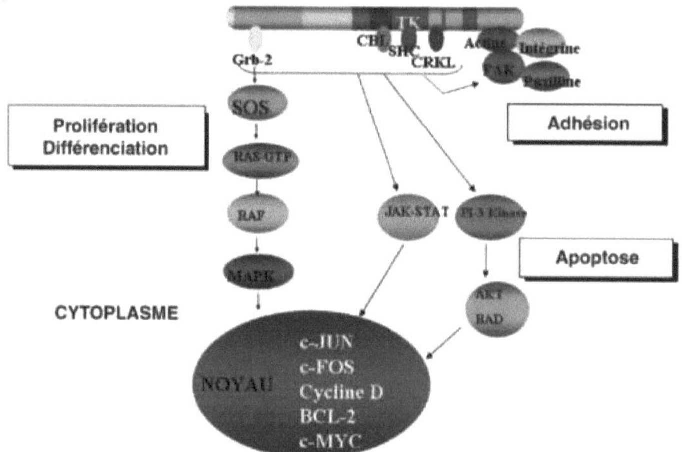

APPENDIX II: Practical treatment plan for a new case of chronic myeloid leukaemia (CML) diagnosed in the chronic phase.

ITK: tyrosine kinase inhibitor; CCyR: complete cytogenetic response.

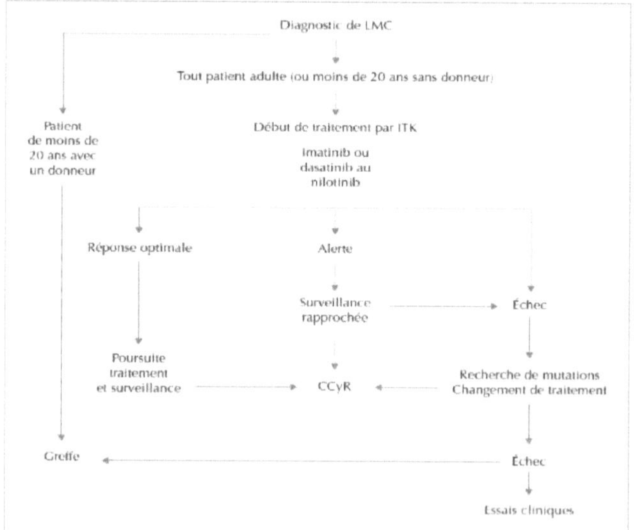

ANNEX III Treatment response criteria and monitoring procedures

Complete hematological	Cytogenetic response (RCy)	Molecular response (MR)

response (CHR)		
-Platelets <450Giga/l - Leukocytes <1 OGiga/l -No myeloma -Basophils < 5 -No splenomegaly	Complete (RCyC) Ph+ 0% Partial (RCyP) Ph+ 1-35% Minor (RCym) Ph+ 3665 Minimal Ph+ 66-95 None Ph+ >95 Major = complete+partial (RCyM)	BCR-ABL/control gene ratio -Major response <0.10% (El) - Deep molecular remission: > RM4 <0.01% (El) > RM4.5<0.0032% (El) > Undetectable: no BCR-ABL gene can be detected.
Follow-up: -At the time of diagnosis -Every 15 days until the RHC is obtained -Then every 3 months	Follow-up: - At diagnosis at 3 and 6 and 2 months until RCyC - After 12 months, if a MMR - If there are any warning signs, repeat all the tests every month - If the disease fails or progresses, cytogenetics, PCR and mutational analysis should be carried out.	Follow-up: -Every 3 months until MMR -Then every 3a 6 months
Mutational analysis: is recommended only if the disease progresses, treatment fails or if there are entertainment signs.		

ANNEX IV:

Information sheet for the diagnosis and follow-up of CML

1) Identification :

Surname, first name: Age: Address Tel:

2) Circumstances of discovery: � Incidental: ⎧ PMS

⎧ Thrombosis Asthenia ⎧ Haemorrhage Hyperleukocytosis ⎧ Past history: Personal: Familial: ⎧ Other :

3) Clinical and biological investigations for diagnostic purposes: ☒ Clinical examination: ⎧ General signs ⎧ Bone pain ⎧ PMS

⎧ Haemorrhage ⎧ Other: ☒ Blood count: ⎧ WBC :

⎧ Hb : ⎧ Platelets : ☒ Blood smear : ⎧ PNN : Blasts : ⎧ Myelimia: Eosinophils: ⎧ Basophils: ☒ MO: Done No Done If yes: Blasts : % ☒ Karyotype: Done No Done ☒ Molecular biology: Done No Done ⎧ BCR/Abl: + - IF + Ratio: % ☒ Uric acid: (if done).

4) Date of diagnosis: Prognostic classification: Sockol :

5) Pre-therapy check-up: Hepatic Glycaemia Renal

DDT :

Hydrea.   Dose: Imatinib Time between dgc and start of TRT: Dose :

7) TRT monitoring :

Complete Hematological	3 MONTHS	YES NO		Dose	

49

Response (CHR)	6 MONTHS	YES		
		NO		

☒ Molecular evaluation :

☒ 6 months :

Yes : BCR/Abel : → ☐ <0,1%   ☐ ≥1%

No: _ Increase in imatinib doses
: _ Switch with a 2nd generation ITK :

➢ **12 mois :** Oui   Non   Si oui   BCR/Abl :<0,1% ☐ ≥1% ☐
➢ **18 mois :** Oui   Non   Si oui   BCR/Abl :<0,1% ☐ ≥1% ☐
➢ **24 mois :** Oui   Non   Si oui   BCR/Abl :<0,1% ☐ ≥1% ☐

8) **Cytogenetic evaluation (karyotype) :** Done No Done

9) **Therapeutic evaluation:** ⎰ Failure: time from start of TRT: ⎰ Relapse: time from remission: _ Haematological. _ Molecular ⎰ Overall survival: (dgc-death) for deceased patients:-date of death: OR -date of last news: ⎰ Progression-free survival (dgc-relapse):-Date of relapse: (PES/EFS)

10) **Tolerance to TRT :** ☒ Clinical complications

☒ Biologically: ⎰ Neutropenia: ⎰ Anemia: ⎰ Thrombocytopenia: ⎰ Liver function tests: AST: ALT: ɣGT: Bilirubin: PAL:

⎰ Blood glucose :

11) **Patients on 2nd generation TKI:** Acutisation: Yes No TRT: if Acutisation :

APPENDIX V: Principle of RT-Q-PCR

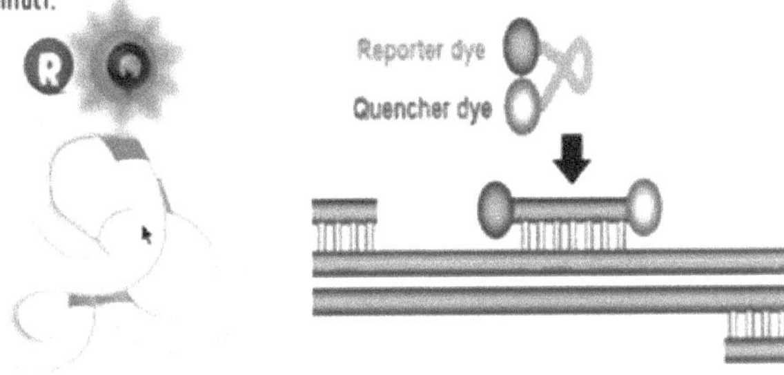

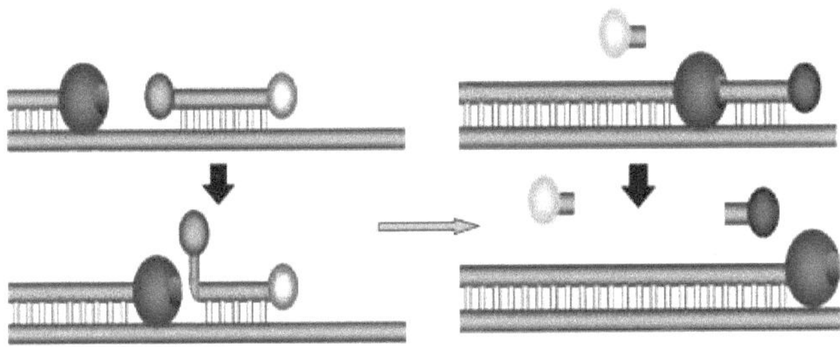

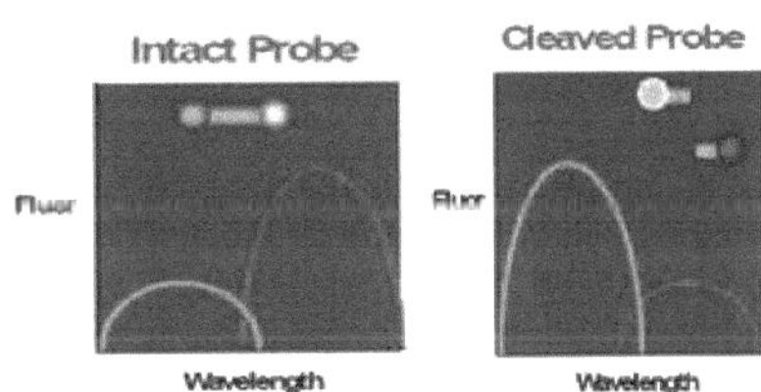

Resume

Molecular monitoring of BCR-ABL transcript levels by quantitative PCR is increasingly used to assess patient response to treatment. This has become of particular interest in the imatinib era when residual disease falls below the detection threshold of conventional cytogenetics. The main objective of our work is to study the revolution of CML by quantifying the BCR/ABL molecular transcript during the therapeutic phase. This is a retrospective, descriptive study of 30 patients followed in the hematology department of the CHU of Tizi Ouzou, at the consultation unit.

Molecular follow-up was carried out for a median period of 24 months (3-34) after the start of treatment. 66.6% of patients had splenomegaly as the predominant clinical sign.

More than half of the study population (56.6%) had a BCR:Abl ratio of 50 to 100% at diagnosis. According to Sokal's prognostic classification, we found a predominance of low risk. Molecular follow-up showed that 70% of patients had MMR with imatinib 400 mg and 20% of patients who had failed imatinib 400 and 600 mg were substituted with a second-generation TKI (nilotinib) with 100% MMR. Quantification of the BCR/Abl ratio showed that 96% of patients on imatinib 400mg were cured. In conclusion, optimisation of treatment, its adjustment and the use of the various TKIs available require biomolecular monitoring of BCR/Abl transmissions from diagnosis onwards in order to assess residual disease.

Key words: CML, TKI, Imatinib, molecular monitoring, BCR/ABL transcript.

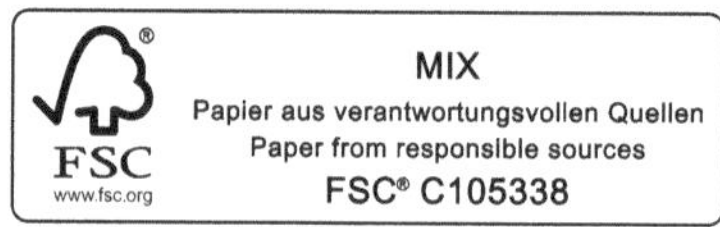

Printed by Books on Demand GmbH, Norderstedt / Germany